BOLD FREEDOM

How to find enough time to live well.
For a happy gut, clear head and more energy.
Inspired by Ayurveda.

Lesley O'Brien
Foreword Amadea Morningstar

©2024 by Lesley O'Brien

DISCLAIMER
This book is not intended to treat, diagnose or prescribe. The information contained herein is in no way to be considered as a substitute for your own good common sense, or as a substitute for a consultation with your health professional.
All rights reserved. No part of this book may be reproduced in any manner whatsoever without written permission except in the case of brief quotations embodied in critical articles or reviews.

Published in Australia
Cover design by Amanda Lu. Designed by Amanda Lu and Silvia Behar.
Edited by Alicia Kacar.
Printed and Distributed by Ingramspark
ISBN: 978-0-646-99245-7

O'Brien, Lesley (Author)
Bold Freedom: How to find enough time to live well. For a happy gut, clear head and more energy.

First printed 2018

Third edition
112 pages

1. SELF-HELP / Self-Management / Time Management
2. HEALTH & FITNESS / Healthy Living & Personal Hygiene
3. MEDICAL / Alternative & Complementary Medicine

To you, adventurous reader.
With special thanks to D, H and the Blosses.

~ Lesley

"Until one is committed, there is hesitancy, the chance to draw back - Concerning all acts of initiative (and creation), there is one elementary truth that ignorance of which kills countless ideas and splendid plans: that the moment one definitely commits oneself, then providence moves too.

All sorts of things occur to help one that would never otherwise have occurred. A whole stream of events issues from the decision, raising in one's favour all manner of unforeseen incidents and meetings and material assistance, which no man could have dreamed would have come his way.

Whatever you can do, or dream you can do, begin it. Boldness has genius, power, and magic in it. Begin it now."

JOHANN WOLFGANG VON GOETHE

CONTENTS

Foreword – by Amadea Morningstar	11
Introduction	17
1. Realign to time	**23**
Begin where you are	24
Big picture possibilities	31
Design doable steps	39
Make time for action	47
2. Reset the scene	**54**
Move the furniture	55
Relationship review	62
3. Know how your body works	**68**
Clear any blocks	69
The daily way	80
4. Enjoy the practice	**94**
Changing direction and troubleshooting	95
Share what you have, rinse and repeat	103
About the Author	109

FOREWORD

Are you interested in taking charge of your health and life with more skill? Are you possibly daunted by what this might mean in practical terms? Hesitate no longer. You can feel better, experience a greater state of wellness, and still have time to enjoy your loved ones and work. Lesley O'Brien's generous passion for healthy sane living is contagious. She details here in Bold Freedom how to take back your life, health and joy. She integrates savvy down to earth life style coaching techniques with the wisdom of Ayurveda. Ayurveda, a 4 – 5,000 year old system of healing originating in India, has become increasingly popular across the globe, because of its effective results. According to one early report from the National Institutes of Health (NIH) in the U.S., a clinical study from UC San Diego School of Medicine showed that in 79% of cases, the health of patients with various chronic diseases improved measurably after Ayurvedic treatment. In a more recent study done by the same university in 2016, a short six days of Ayurvedic life style changes resulted in measurable improvements in inflammatory markers for participants. Learn how you can easily apply Ayurvedic principles of healing in your own life with Bold Freedom.

Lesley invites you to discover how to find enough time to live well, with a clear head, more energy, and a happy gut. Planning ahead, you track your progress, learn how to use your intuition to make wise choices and your consistency to achieve your goals. This is a system that empowers you and is designed to fit your life style. The author's upbeat positive attitude inspires people interested in deeper wellness to "get on board!".

One apparent mission in this life for me has been to introduce ordinary people (that is, any of us) to the deeper esoteric healing practices of India and Tibet. They are often a lot simpler to experience and apply than one might suspect. I have especially appreciated how Ayurveda opens to the whole person, not just our physical selves, yet also our energetic, emotional, intellectual, and spiritual selves. Practicing a system of healing that opens to all of who we are has been a relief for me personally. To offer a bridge from what Ayurveda has to share to a Western audience takes interest and some skill. I share this pleasure and interest with Lesley O'Brien. While Ayurveda is effective, it can also be intimidating. Lesley makes this ancient science something you can simply apply for yourself. For this, I honour her.

Bold Freedom shows you how to apply Ayurveda skilfully in your own life. It's one thing to know what you need to do, yet another thing to actually be able to do it. The author introduces you to Ayurveda with practices of simple clear planning, nothing fancy. Using Brian Moran's 12-week year, based on effective business planning, she details how to align your daily routine with nature, one season at a time. This planning is essential for success in applying these new and often exciting ideas. Unabashedly Western in her outlook, Lesley defines *ama*, undigested toxic wastes, in broad terms appropriate for the 21st century. It's not just the food you eat that can create sticky waste in your life, it's also the undigested emotions and sensory stimulation. With this in mind, one of the short tips for wellness offered here is a "Digital Detox".

O'Brien is an ardent and effective life style coach. She wants you to succeed, and her methods are practical. She invites you to take time and create space for your intentions. She introduces you to how your body works from an Ayurvedic perspective. She offers multiple ways of making skilful choices. One support is her clear, useful self-care tips, such as "create triggers". What is a trigger? Something that will remind you to do what you want (and have planned) to do. A favourite trigger that I use in my Ayurvedic self-care practice with clients is the recommendation to put on tennis/walking/hiking shoes, whatever you like. Once you've got them on your feet, you invite yourself to go for a walk. It's about working with momentum.

The author is realistic about the world that we readers live in, one in which you need to make a living, find healthy ways to eat and get along with your boss and loved ones.
This down to earth expertise is reflected in the case studies of real people dealing with common problems. They are inspiring in their ability to remind us that it is possible to make small changes, and these small skilful win-win solutions can make a big difference in one's health and wellbeing.

| Foreword

Bold Freedom offers a rather radical take on Ayurveda. Rather than working with the biological energies known as the doshas, its essential first planning step relates to nature and the five elements. You are invited to assess where you are in five key areas of your life that are then related to the elements: your environment (ether), your time (air), your energy (fire), your abilities (water), and your finances (earth). It works.

It could be interesting to relate the time-honoured Ayurvedic qualities of the mind, the *Mahagunas* of sattva, rajas and *tamas*, more to this planning process, particularly in light of recent developments in Western science related to the autonomic nervous system. Stephen W. Porges and other researchers have described three basic ANS states in what is called Polyvagal Theory (PVT). These are automatic functions of the nervous system, yet they can be influenced by conscious awareness. In the first state, ventral vagal complex (VVC) you feel comfortable inside yourself and within your environment. You feel connected and secure with those you are with, part of parasympathetic nervous system function. This experience sounds very much like the loving, neutral, secure state of *sattva*. The second state, related to the sympathetic nervous system (SNS), mediates "fight or flight" responses and tends to dominate when you're pushing to complete a project or point of view, like *rajas*, warm, pushy, assertive. The third state, dorsal vagal complex (DVC) relates to the protective state of immobilization, when one tends to shut down in the face of stress. (Effective DVC function also is associated with the parasympathetic nervous system's "rest and digest" processes.) Tamas, the third of the mahagunas, embodies constriction, slowdown, like DVC. The exciting part of working with either Polyvagal theory or the Mahagunas is that you can consciously shift your behaviour in response to another's nervous system. If a client or loved one is accelerating into a panicked, rajasic, sympathetic dominant state, you can extend compassion and work to connect, evoking sattva and a VVC state. You can use this awareness yourself in applying the *Bold Freedom* methods of wellness. If you get pushy or overly judgmental with yourself, you can step in with some deep breaths (see Lesley's self-care tips for specific hints) and shift to a more sattvic state.

It doesn't need to be rocket science. Lesley breaks down *Dinacharya*, Ayurvedic life style routines into simple one-word bites. Here they are for a Morning Routine:

pause – hydrate – eliminate – refresh – oil – move – breathe - eat. No problem!

It's important to remember that Ayurveda works with opposites for healing. If we're moving into a warm season, we'll create ways to cool ourselves down. If the environment is dry, then oil, whether in food or as a rub, is important. We naturally tend toward this balancing flow, it's one of those places where our common sense and Ayurveda easily come into alignment.

Food cravings are a popular topic of conversation in many classes I lead. It's interesting to look at Ayurveda's approach to these. In Ayurveda *Samprapti*, there are six stages of how disease can develop (or not). The first four of these are completely under Western medicine's radar, that is, it's not until the fifth stage of disease in Ayurveda that an obvious illness actually appears. The six stages are: accumulation (of a subtle imbalance or energy), provocation, spread, deposition, manifestation (when a disease can be seen), and differentiation. Interestingly, when healthy energy first starts going awry for us, our natural instincts are to counterbalance the problem. We're chilly inside, we naturally gravitate toward healthy hot drinks and foods, "healthy cravings". Yet if an imbalance gets deeper, our cravings flip to "unhealthy" ones. We've run around too much, we're exhausted, yet paradoxically we'll pace the house and eat junk food. A deeper understanding of the doshas can help us understand and work with these states.

Yet intuitively we often know what we need to do for ourselves. We may not need to know all the specific effects white sugar has on our doshas and *dhatus* (essential tissues) to know that we'd feel better taking in less of it. Here's where Lesley's plan of Bold Freedom comes in, with myriad supports for actually doing what you want to do.
For a sound, practical approach to integrating Ayurveda into your daily life, thereby increasing your chances for good health, sound mind and a happy belly, enjoy this book.

May whatever happiness and health results from these efforts be used with compassion and wisdom to help everyone in the ways only we can do as individuals,
With respect and gladness,

Amadea Morningstar, BS (nutrition) MA (counselling) RPE (polarity therapy) RYT (yoga)

Author of Easy Healing Drinks from the Wisdom of Ayurveda and "Ayurveda: Relevance in Culture Care" with Joanna B. Maxwell in *Leininger's Transcultural Nursing* (2018)

INTRODUCTION

If you've found this book (or this book has found you), you're clearly passionate about wellbeing. You want to create your healthiest body, your happiest mind, and live your best life. These are simple yet noble goals. However, like most people, you're probably confused about how to reach them.

With the huge number of resources available, it's easy to feel overwhelmed when it comes to health. You can read, watch and listen to hours of content, but nothing ever seems to stick. How many times have you implemented a plan, but forgotten to track your progress? Or tried to follow a wellness program, which just didn't suit your lifestyle? Perhaps you suffer from "shiny object syndrome" (a common phenomenon in our modern world). When your body is sick and flaring up, it's tempting to follow the latest trend. But putting out spot fires is exhausting, and it rarely leads to long-term results.

The good news is, there is a way to optimise your body and nourish your soul. It's effective, flexible, and easy to follow. In fact, you already know what to do. You see, there are two key ingredients in the recipe for wellbeing – intuition and consistency. Regardless of where you're currently at, I believe you know what your body needs. You just don't do it consistently enough to get the results you want. That's where Ayurveda comes in.

Ayurveda is a 4,000-year old system of traditional medicine, originating in India. It's the oldest recorded medical system and was developed from ancient seers observing nature. The word Ayurveda is composed of two Sanskrit words – "ayur" meaning life, and "veda" meaning knowledge. It translates to "the knowledge of healthy living" and is based on the understanding that you are created from the five elements of life – Earth, Water, Fire, Wind and Space. Ayurveda strengthens your body and mind. It puts you in harmony with the environment, allowing you to respond to all of life's challenges – physical, emotional and spiritual – with grace and poise.

Unlike some other health systems, Ayurveda doesn't take a "one size fits all approach". The guiding principles of Ayurveda work best when they're tailored to you individually. Ayurveda is adaptable and pragmatic, which is one of many reasons why it's still used today in hundreds of hospitals and clinics around the world. Ayurveda starts with you – and if you're looking for a simple, effective solution to wellbeing, start with Ayurveda.

When you take the Ayurvedic approach, you'll notice how easy it becomes to manage your health, prevent illness and increase your energy. Because Ayurveda understands that the foundational principles of healthy living need to adjust with the natural rhythms of the seasons and individuals, it allows space for creativity and new opportunities to arise. Imagine having a system that empowers you and fits your lifestyle. One that allows you to take control of your health, without following the latest fads, or spending a fortune on superfoods. Imagine if feeling well was no longer a struggle, but a natural part of every day. It's all possible with Ayurveda.

With Ayurveda you can design a way of life you can consistently tap into, that's deeply aligned with your unique body, and that makes sense to you at any given moment. This simple yet powerful system asks you to listen to your body, trust your intuition, take what serves you, and ditch the rest – because no one knows your body better than you do. When you do this, wellbeing will follow. You'll no longer feel frazzled or overwhelmed – and you'll never "fail" at another plan. Living well will become simple, natural and enjoyable. How liberating does that sound?

"We can't solve problems if we use the same kind of thinking we used when we created them."
ALBERT EINSTEIN

It's time to choose. You can continue struggling down the same beaten path, or you can listen to the voice deep inside that's beckoning you to show up for your own health. Let go of the old ways that no longer serve you and embrace the life-changing power of Ayurveda. Just like any lifestyle change, it's normal to feel scared or tentative. However, once you let go of your fears and limiting beliefs, the rewards from Ayurveda will be amazing – for you, those around you, and the environment. When you're gentle and strong from living true, you'll be a support and inspiration for other people, while making positive health choices that benefit the planet.

Now is your time. And, if not now, when? As the Earth changes with environmental, political and economic impacts, there's never been a better time to take charge of your life. Instead of simply surviving, be one of the people who thrives. Someone who can figure out ways to stay happy and healthy – who enjoys optimum health and abundant energy, and who glows from the inside out. The alternative is to stay as you are, but is that working for you? What would your life look like in five years if you didn't change anything?

Everything you need is already inside you. This book will teach you how to unlock it. Be brave. Be liberated. Be boldly free with Ayurveda.

HOW TO USE THIS BOOK

Without a plan, it's easy to revert to old habits. The Bold Freedom method helps you establish positive daily habits that take you where you want to be. As these healthy habits form, you'll feel better in your body, stronger in your mind, and happier in your heart. With the flexible Bold Freedom method, you are always in control. You choose how deep and how fast you want to go, and which paths you want to take.

In terms of how the process is structured, Bold Freedom is based on Brian Moran's "12-week year" method. This method breaks the year into four quarters with regular review and reset periods. Here's how it looks:

Q1: Jan, Feb, Mar (in the last week of March review Q1 and get ready for Q2)

Q2: Apr, May, Jun (in the last week of June review Q2 and get ready for Q3)

Q3: Jul, Aug, Sep (in the last week of September review Q3 and get ready for Q4)

Q4: Oct, Nov, Dec (in the last week of December review Q3 and prepare for Q1 of the new year)

Why the 12-week year? I'm glad you asked! Brian created the 12-week year after observing that businesses perform at their peak in the last quarter. They fluff around for the first three quarters, then surge home to meet their goals. After implementing this technique in my online health practice, I realised how effective it was. I also saw its potential to help patients reach their health goals. I trialled it out with my team and the results were incredible. I know your results will be incredible too.

Aside from being remarkably motivating, the best thing about the 12-week year method is that it provides space to pivot and tweak. As you progress through your Bold Freedom journey, you'll find regular check-in and reset points. These allow you to assess how you're feeling, what's working and what's not. With this method, you can design a plan that perfectly fits your lifestyle, a plan you love, that loves you back – and sits well with your current resources, including time, budget and energy.

If you're feeling daunted, don't be. One year is a long time, but bold Freedom takes you step-by-step through the vast possibilities of Ayurveda. You'll be regularly guided to "ask the question behind the question", as it's here that freedom resides. To help you get the most from this book (and from the Bold Freedom method) here are some simple tips.

- Read the chapters in order, then begin the method from Step 1. This will allow you to get a big picture view before you begin. Alternatively, you can dive into the chapter that interests you most. Read the book in any order you like but begin the method from Step 1.

- Bold Freedom works best when aligned to the four quarters of the calendar year, but that doesn't mean you can't start now. Read the book, draw up your calendar and have a practice run. This will mean you're ready to kick off in either January, April, July or October (whichever comes first).

- Have a notebook handy as your read. Most sections of Bold Freedom will include small note taking activities. These are designed to help you get clear on your goals and complete the larger activities.

- Just like the seasons cycle and change, so should you. Review and reset four times a year (in the last week of March, June, September and December), so you're perfectly poised for the next twelve weeks.

- Be brave and approach Bold Freedom with an open heart and open mind. You may discover that you're attached to certain habits or stressors, simply because they're so familiar. It can be scary to confront ingrained beliefs, but freedom awaits on the other side!

After seven years of research and two years of testing, I'm so proud to bring you the Bold Freedom method. This book has been influenced by the many people who I've learnt from plus the people I help through my Ayurvedic practice. I'm thankful to everyone who's guided me on my own journey to Bold Freedom – and I'm honoured to guide you through yours.

Yours in health and happiness,
Lesley O'Brien

THE BOLD FREEDOM METHOD

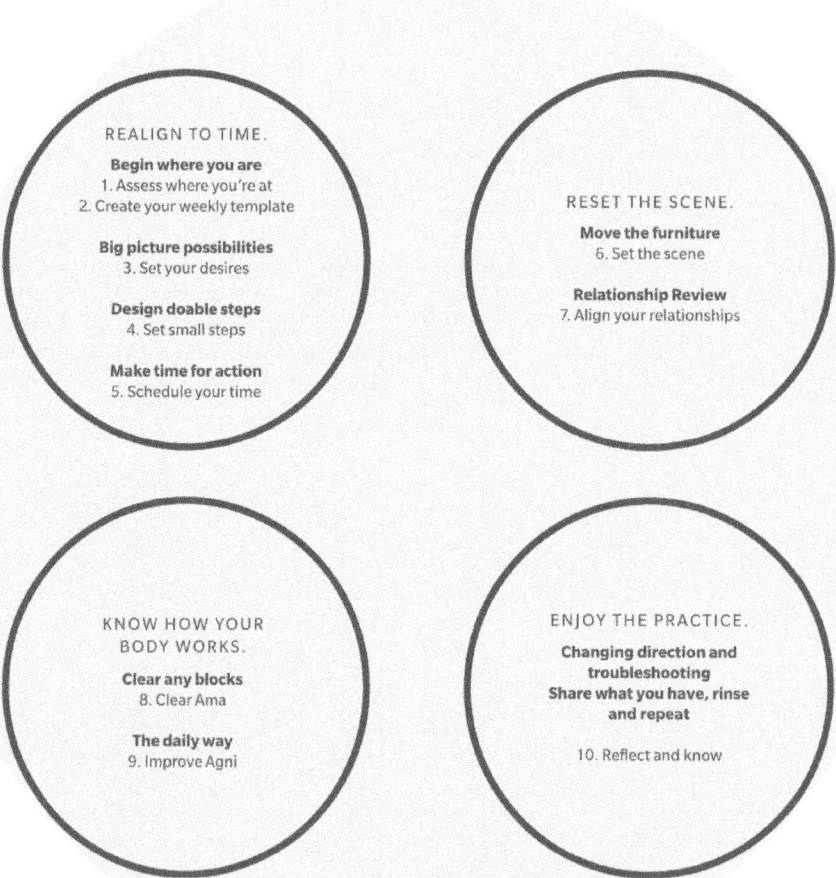

ONE: REALIGN TO TIME

BEGIN WHERE YOU ARE

Time will start to bend in your favour as soon as you focus on living your truth.

Have you ever sat down and mapped out your time before beginning to pave the way ahead? Too many times we launch into action, hoping to reach an outcome sooner. But failing to plan is planning to fail. Short cuts simply don't lead to success. Plus, living life on fast forward, in a perpetual state of stress, wreaks havoc with your body and mind.

This chapter is all about slowing down and taking time to plan for success. It's about getting clear on what you REALLY want, then designing a blueprint to get you there. And not a "one size fits all" blueprint. One that's created just for you, that works with your time and resources. Just like there are many treatments for an upset gut, there are many ways to create a plan. However, to ensure you experience great results, your plan should include these key components:
- A clear starting point
- Your true "why?" or motivation (dig deep for this one)
- The current resources you have at your disposal
- Areas that may need support (including how and where you will get it)
- Troubleshooting solutions for "off" days

Bold Freedom ensures you tick all these boxes, giving you the best possible chance of success. This is a twelve-month journey, but you only need to take things one day at a time. After all, life is busy. It's so easy to get caught up in mundane activities that time becomes a dull blur. Bold Freedom recognises this. It also recognises that, when you're in this blurry state, old habits take over. This book will teach you how to slow down, keep focused and stay in the present moment so you don't bounce back to default mode.

~

One thing to remember as you go through this journey is that you are in control. Regardless of what's going on in your life, there are always choices. You can usually choose what you eat, how you move your body, and what you give attention to. Some days will be harder than others. There's no doubt about that. But when these days strike, perspective, gratitude and a great attitude will get you through. You'll be surprised at how adaptable you can be when you truly commit and consistently show up.

Think about how others adapt. For some people, the only choice is survival and the attitude they bring to it. When I lived in Asia, I mingled with the locals, learnt the languages and made friends. I committed to this new environment. I chose to immerse myself in the culture. Every day, I made the effort to show up, even when it was challenging. Instead of feeling isolated and overwhelmed, I had an absolute ball!

Bold Freedom asks you to commit to a new way of living. It asks you to CHOOSE health and happiness. It also asks you to be selfish, because this journey is about YOU. How many times have you said, 'the office needs me' or 'the family needs me', as if they wouldn't manage without you? Believe it or not, the way to assume real health is to fill your own cup first. Make time and space for things you love. It's only when you are healthy and happy, that you can share your unique gifts with the world. At first, it might feel a little indulgent, but trust that it's true kindness in action.

When you choose to live in a way that nourishes your soul, life's possibilities are endless. Time on Earth is finite, so give each day the attention it deserves. When you direct your energy to the right places, you'll be amazed at how the universe responds. You'll soon find yourself with more time and energy to do things you love, because that's what you're focusing on. This enjoyment is essential in your journey to wellbeing. The concentration sector of your brain is situated right near the pleasure centre, so the happier you are, the more motivated you'll be!

Plus, when you make time to do things that make your heart sing, everything else seems a little bit easier. You begin to approach mundane life activities with a sense of calmness and gratitude. Tasks like cleaning or grocery shopping become enjoyable, because you know those things keep your space and body well. And because you've made time somewhere else in your day to do something important. Even when things are imposed on you, like a work deadline or family emergency, you'll learn to accept them with grace and ease as you implement the Bold Freedom method. Things you may have seen as a burden will become "just stuff" and life will become a delightful game. Gratitude will replace resentment. Imagine how freeing that could feel?

This gratitude, when it comes, will come without judgement or strings attached. Think about what sometimes happens when you actively try to "do" gratitude. Have you ever criticised someone for being "ungrateful" when they complain about something small? We're all guilty of this behaviour, but it doesn't help our own gratitude practice. Instead, it keeps us comparing ourselves to others, disconnects us from our community, and forces us to look outward rather than reflect inward. Just like Ayurveda, gratitude begins with you. As you move through this book, you'll become more in tune with your inner self. You'll learn to face your own challenges and make them easeful, no matter how confronting they seem. Then, when you observe others, you'll be more accepting of their story. It will be easy to offer a listening ear without having to say a word. Again, this is kindness in action.

~

Perspective, gratitude and a positive attitude are your tickets to Bold Freedom. But, of course, there'll be roadblocks along the way. As you plan and implement the Bold Freedom method, you're bound to bump into some old friends – like fear, impatience and procrastination. Allow them to visit. Sit with them. You might even spend some time entertaining them, but the conversation will be much different to what it's been in the past. Instead of succumbing to negative feelings, you'll actually notice them and be better prepared to send them on their merry way.

If you can, find new friends to support you on your journey. A common trait of successful people is that they surround themselves with like-minded people. The more support you have, the faster you'll reach your destination

– and the more fun you'll have along the way. This idea has been reinforced many times in my own life. One thing I've learnt from people from all walks of life (especially travelling overseas) is that community comes from a sense of belonging. You're so much more likely to show up when people are supporting and expecting you. With that in mind, why not ask a family member, friend or colleague to join you on your journey to Bold Freedom? Your plans and goals will be different, but you'll face similar challenges along the way.

If you're called to travel the road alone, that's absolutely fine. But you'll need to be your own best friend. That means acknowledging where you are now and treating yourself with kindness and compassion. Accept your current state, no matter how dire it seems. Embrace it. Every step you take will bring you closer to Bold Freedom. The important thing is that you begin. So, let's begin right now by looking at where you're at.

STEP 1 ASSESS WHERE YOU'RE AT
Think about each of the areas below and write down how you feel. Do you feel fine or is there room for improvement? Do you feel lacking or blocked in any way?

- Your environment – this is the element of Ether manifesting. Everything happens in space!
- Your time – closely related to the element of Air and your own life-giving breath.
- Your energy – this correlates with your life's purpose and is linked to element of Fire.
- Your abilities – do you flow through life with clarity and ease like the element of Water?
- Your finances – your body and the element of Earth reside around this stable area.

Energy can come from any of these resources, but the aim is to keep them all balanced. If you feel lacking in time, take a few deep breaths and focus on air. Similarly, if you're struggling with low energy, it could be because you're not following your intuition. Where is your nervous system at now? Did you note that you feel blocked in your environment? Recognise what that means for you. It could be something relational, or simply that there's not enough physical space in your living room!

No matter where you're at, congratulations for being brave. Taking stock of your current situation is the first step to Bold Freedom. There's no need to worry about what you "should" be doing, or where you think you've gone wrong. It's fine to acknowledge that something's hard, or that some things need to change, but try not to dwell on the negative. Instead, think about how you'd prefer things to look. Where would you like to be one year from now? What resources do you have already, and what do you need to move forward? Once you have a clear goal and vision, you can work backwards to create a plan. We'll start with that in Step 2. For now, all you need to know is that you're perfectly lovely just as you are.

STEP 2 CREATE YOUR WEEKLY TEMPLATE

Have you ever noticed how you add to your stress by searching frantically for the latest learnings and treatments? There are millions of resources on the market, but the best investment you can make is trust in your own ability. When it comes to nourishing your body, you know what to do. You just need to do it consistently.

In a moment you'll use your calendar to look more closely at where you're at. The aim is to find out how you spend your time, assess your current habits, and make space for new ones. As you go through this exercise, you'll likely discover you have a lot of resources you can tap into. You may find you have more spare time than you think. Or maybe you won't. Either way, it will be glaringly obvious when you see it in black and white. And whatever time you have available, rest assured we can work around it. That's the beauty of bold freedom. Let's dive right in.

- **Get a hard copy weekly calendar.** You can print out a weekly calendar or draw one up on a sheet of paper. An offline calendar is preferable to an online calendar for setting goals. In fact, when you physically write down your goals on paper, you're ten times more likely to follow through. I learnt this during an allied health coaching session conducted by psychologists. In their studies, they found most patients failed to follow through on practitioner's recommendations unless they were written down. These patients knew exactly what to do, but they failed to plan – so they planned to fail. Grab your calendar now.

- **Add in essential commitments.** Create blocks in your calendar for non-negotiable things in your week. If your work hours are 9am to 5pm, Monday to Friday, block that time out. Do the same with all other commitments, like school, Uni or appointments. Do this for the entire week. What you're creating here is a weekly template. As well as identifying your available time, this exercise is a perfect opportunity for self-reflection. If you're blocking out large chunks of time for work, ask yourself what you're really working for? Is it for money? If so, that's great. Is it because you love your job? That is brilliant too. Understanding the 'why?' behind 'what' you do is a big part of this process.

- **Add in everything else.** Now block out time for everything else you usually do in your week. Perhaps you go to the gym every morning, walk the dog or call your mum. You might have a ritual of cleaning your car every Saturday morning. Or doing the groceries on Wednesday night. Include everything you can think of, including time for daily meals. And remember to leave some white space. The last thing you want is to be flying from one activity to another without a second to spare in between. I recommend leaving a minimum of five minutes between each task. A little more if you have time.

- **Take a good hard look at your habits.** Do you notice any trends? You may have plenty of healthy habits, but there's likely room for improvement too. When you look at the breakdown of your week, you might notice how one bad habit can lead to another. For example, you may let your morning exercise slip when you don't allow enough time in the day. Then, because you're so stretched, you eat your evening meal late. You sleep poorly and wake up the next day feeling tired and heavy. You then skip your workout the following day because you don't have the energy. And on the story goes. If you notice patterns like this, write them down in your notepad.

~

Congratulations! You've completed your first weekly template. Well done for staring time in the face. If you've never done something like this before, you might be shocked by the results – for better or for worse. Seeing your week in black and white might be confronting, but ignorance doesn't equal bliss. In Bold Freedom, knowledge is power – and you've empowered yourself with the knowledge to move forward. Plus, behavioural science shows that 40% of what we do is determined by habit. Once you replace unhealthy habits with healthy ones, you'll put your wellbeing on autopilot!

- **Make a note:** If you're feeling really overwhelmed, grab another piece of paper and write down your emotions. Don't be too hard on yourself. Remember, to break through, you have to break down. Things will change when you do.

Pledge to make your health and happiness a priority from this day forward. Trust that this process takes practice and give yourself time to grow. Wherever you are right now is exactly where you're supposed to be. In the following chapters you'll set your goals and create a personalised plan of attack. You can read ahead about what's to come, but there's no need to take action just yet. Your only job at this moment is to hold space for change to begin. Lean into this transformative process. The future looks delightfully bright!

~

Self-care tip you can try today - A life-giving lunch.
The gut and the head are closely connected. If you want to have a clear mind and sharp senses, eat the "elements of life" at lunch time. How does your lunch feel, look and taste? Does it contain the elements of air, mostly water and some substance? Is it warm and made of wholefoods? Eating clean, nutrient dense food is easier on your entire system, especially your digestive system. Healthy foods encourage your body to detox and prevent the build-up of toxic substances, called "Ama" in Ayurveda. Ama can manifest in many forms, from mucous to emotions, and is often formed through poor dietary habits and low digestive fire. If you want to do your body one favour today, start with a life-giving lunch. We'll talk more about lunch in the next chapter – and more about Ama in the subsequent sections.

BIG PICTURE POSSIBILITIES

The definition of success is different for everyone. In this chapter, you'll get clear on what success looks like to you. You may think you already know but be prepared to surprise yourself. Sometimes what you THINK you want is much different to what you REALLY want. Get ready to go deep!

For many people, a helpful way to think about success is in terms of "flow" and integrity. Think about how many different roles you play in your week. You could be a parent, worker, athlete, friend, shopper, cleaner, cook, artist or patient – and anything in between. Success doesn't depend on how many hours you spend in these roles, but rather how seamlessly you flow between them. This is what Simon Sinek defined as true work-life balance. Can you switch effortlessly from one role to the next? Are your roles aligned to your core values? Do you enjoy how you spend your time? This stuff really matters!

Make a note: Take a moment to think about your own definition of success. Write down specifically what it means to you. Is it about living in integrity with your values, or achieving flow, as described above? Or is it about reaching a more specific goal, such as earning a set amount of money, living a certain type of lifestyle, or being recognised by your peers? Write it down in as much detail as you can. Be curious and daring when you do this exercise. And be careful what you wish for. The things you focus on do manifest and they don't always look how you expect.

~

The Bold Freedom method will help you align the next chapter of your life with your definition of success, whatever that looks like. The aim is to balance the five key areas – environment, time, energy, abilities and finances – so they support your spirit and core values. But what are your core values? Have you ever taken time to think about this? Getting clear on your core values is the foundation of good health and happiness. When you know what your priorities are, you can focus on giving them more attention – and ignore the things that aren't as important. This will help you enormously when it comes to completing your plan. Let's do it right now.

- **Make a note:** Create a list of your priorities. What's your number one priority? The most important thing in your life? Is it providing for your family? Your status at work? Money? Spending time with friends? Keeping fit? List your top ten priorities in order. There is no right or wrong answer. Everyone's list will look different.

Seeing your priorities on paper will not only help you make the most of your time and energy, it will help you understand where your values come from. Why do you think the way you do? What circumstances have made you the delightfully unique person you've grown to become? Which thoughts, factors and beliefs have shaped your journey? Are they still serving you?

~

You may not have considered this before, but your priorities and values are shaped by your ancestry. Think about your family. What traits, experiences and struggles stand out? Did your father or mother experience any trauma in their lives? Did your grandparents suffer through famine or war? Was there a significant tragedy or loss in your family? In Ayurveda, we believe the experiences of your ancestors are stored in your DNA. Emotions are captured in cell memory and passed down through generations. Your unique view of the world is influenced by these emotions – some positive, some negative. If there's been significant trauma in your family, it could impact the way you approach life. Your approach to food, money, relationships, status. All these things are influenced.

Don't feel alarmed by this idea. While your ancestry shapes who you've become, it doesn't define who you are. Use this knowledge about your past as power. When you understand why you tend towards certain habits or thought patterns, you can control them with greater ease. Like everything in the Bold Freedom method, this process takes patience. It takes time for stories to unravel, be learnt from and let go. Simply recognise your ancestral patterns and revisit the stories as you reflect through your journey. Think about the things you did, said or ate at the end of each day, and how those things left you feeling. Observe your thoughts and actions. How might they connect to your past? Be curious and commit, but never judge yourself harshly. Remember, you are your own best friend.

~

As you observe your feelings and behaviours from a place of compassion, you'll may start to notice patterns. You might notice that you have more energy when you go to bed early, or when you start your day with some gentle stretching. On the other hand, you may find your body reacts poorly to certain foods, or that you hit a slump in the mid-afternoon. Simply notice what you notice. Then aim to do more of what makes you feel better. One day at a time.

One thing that will help, if your schedule allows, is aligning your daily routine with nature. The more you align to the natural rhythms of how you were designed as a primate, the more vibrant you will feel. That means avoiding eating after dark, going to sleep by 10pm, drinking water when you wake up, and plugging in to internal desires. As your body syncs with Mother Nature, you'll feel better equipped to handle whatever life throws at you. Courage and strength will become natural responses. Your mind will be sharp, your head will be clear, and you'll react with poise in all situations. Your natural instincts will kick in.

Think about a time when you've responded naturally to a situation. Like when someone has injured themselves and you've rushed to their aid. Or when you've needed to evacuate a building. In those moments, you don't ask questions. You know intrinsically what to do. Sure, you may feel afraid, but you don't allow fear to take control. Now think about what could happen in those situations if you DID let fear take the wheel. When you overthink a situation, your internal dialogue takes over. This disrupts your natural heart-head response. You operate from a place of fear, which is where confusion, overwhelm and poor choices creep in.

Fear is an instinct designed to protect you. It has a very important role, but only when you really need it. If you're operating on fear, your body gets confused about the messages it's receiving. Your nervous system becomes stressed and frazzled and it's impossible to think clearly. Think about your wellbeing journey. Have you been operating out of fear? Bouncing from one fad to the next, desperately seeking a magic solution? If so, your fear response could be a natural part of your DNA. Accept that it's part of your history, but it doesn't have to be part of your future.

~

Provided you show up for this journey, your future looks incredibly bright! Bold Freedom will teach you how to tap into your intuition, override thoughts and habits that no longer serve you, and approach life with grace and ease. Using the flexible principles of Ayurveda, you'll map out a plan that's perfectly aligned to your values and priorities. So, when you achieve success, it will look exactly how you imagined. But first, two quick tips to settle your nervous system and get you firing on all the right cylinders.

Self-care tip you can try today - A night time routine.
How well do you prepare for a good night's sleep? Are you guilty of scrolling through your phone or watching TV in bed? A night time routine is so important to help your body heal. By reducing the stimulation through your eyes, ears, nose and taste buds, your mind can focus on inward processes – like preparing to repair and cleanse your body naturally while you sleep. Try this night time routine and see how you feel the next day.

Begin winding down around 8:30 pm. First, turn off all devices and screens and dim the lights. Try to tap into the present moment, without worrying about tomorrow. Instead of thinking about what will you wear or mentally preparing for work, focus on what you did today. What made you feel good? Was it a healthy lunch? A walk in the park? Make a mental note to incorporate more of that in your week.

At 9.00pm, go to the bathroom, brush your teeth and get ready for bed. Rub your feet, with or without oil, gently activating every joint in your toes. Rub over the arch of your foot, from toes to heal, and the arc across the bottom of your toes. Through touching your feet and intuitively applying reflexology, you create gentle triggers for bodily processes. If you find this more stimulating than soothing, you can try this in the morning instead. Your body loves to experiment and expand in a safe, consistent environment. You're here to gain experience over time.

Self-care tip you can try today - Digital detox.
Have you ever left your phone at home and realised you didn't miss it that much? Mobile phones are such a huge part of modern lifestyle, but you can get too much of a good thing. The constant ringing, beeping and notifications can wreak havoc with your nervous system, putting you in a perpetual state of high alert. Try leaving your phone at home and take back time in your day. If a whole day sounds too daunting, start with a couple of hours. At the very least, put your phone on silent and track your time on social media. Once you get used to ignoring your phone, you'll notice your nervous system settle. You'll also find that most things can wait for your attention. You don't need to respond instantly. That is a fear-based response!

~

STEP 3 SET YOUR DESIRES
Now you're clear on your values and priorities, it's time to set your yearly goal and the sub-goals around it. This is the exciting part! Profound positive change is coming – and it all starts with a clear vision. Successful people from all walks of life, including sport, business, wellness and more, use reverse-engineering to bring goals to life. They begin with a vision then work backwards, designing a plan to get them there. This is exactly what you will doing, using the principles of Ayurveda.

Unlike some goal setting tools that don't account for your individual lifestyle (like the fact you have a day job, or you lack skills and resources to get started), Bold Freedom begins wherever you are. It recognises that you have a good heart and a strong mind – and that you know what's best for your body. When mapping out your goals for the next twelve months, start with the resources you already have. If there's something more you want or need, you can add this to your five-year plan. It's good to have longer-term goals and look at the bigger picture, but trust that you can build on what you've already got. Your resources (whatever they are) are sufficient and abundant.

In the same way that you don't need to HAVE everything right now, you don't need to DO everything right now. Sometimes the smallest steps lead to the biggest change – and every step in the Bold Freedom method is a bridge to something bigger. So, if you need to take some baby steps towards one giant leap, give yourself permission to do that. Say, for example, you want to start a music career. You may need to get a day job to pay for music lessons or purchase an instrument. Great things take time to develop. However, when you have a plan that's based on passion, success is almost a certainty. Of course, you want to reach the destination, but you also want to enjoy the journey, right? Let's begin setting your goals.

1. **Write down all your SMART goals.** Include everything you want to achieve within the next 12 months in as much detail as possible. Include as many goals as you like, but make sure they are SMART goals. SMART stands for Specific, Measurable, Achievable, Realistic and Timely. Some examples I've heard from patients include paying off credit card debts so they can stop stressing about money, or saving enough to travel to a dream destination. These goals have feelings associated to them. They are measurable. With SMART goals, you know when you reach them. Some examples of non-SMART goals include sleeping better or reducing pain. These are great goals, but how can you measure them? If your goal is to reduce pain, turn it into a SMART goal. Rate your pain now on a scale of 1-10. That way you can track your progress week to week and measure how much your pain reduces.

2. **Define your overarching goal.** Look at all the goals you've written down and use them to define your big annual goal for the year. What's the one feeling or big thing you want to accomplish in the next twelve months? This goal will probably be related to a feeling of wellness or health. This is your deepest desire. An example might be to love and accept yourself unconditionally. Or to let go of past experiences. By simply honouring and writing your deepest desire down, you already begin to make it real. If twelve months feels too far away, it's OK to shorten the time. You might choose your birthday or New Year's Day.

3. **Get clear on your "why?" Why do you want to achieve this goal? Why is it so important? This requires some deep digging.** You may need to ask "why?" many times before you uncover the real answer. Here's an example of how this might sound: Why do I want to lose weight? So I can fit into smaller clothes? Why do I want to fit into smaller clothes? So I can feel more confident. Why do I want to feel more confident? So I can feel

happier in myself. Why do I want to feel happier in myself? So I can be a better parent to my children. Bingo! In this example, weight loss is the goal, but being a better parent is the "why?" Try it and see how you go.

4. **Visualise achieving your goal.** Imagine how your life will be when your goal becomes a reality. How will you feel? What will life look like? What exactly will change? Write down words that signify this in as much detail as possible.

5. **Break your big goal into sub-goals.** The kindest thing you can do for yourself and those around you is to work gradually at your own pace. Breaking big goals down into smaller chunks makes them much more achievable. Let's do that now. Take your big overarching goal and split it into sub-goals. For example, using the weight loss example described above, a 20kg weight loss goal could be broken down into four 5kg sub-goals.

6. **Review to do no harm.** Even though goal setting is an individual process, it's connected to the world at large. If you honestly tap into your heart's desires, the goals you set will be well intentioned. They will have a shared spirit of goodness and they will not hurt or inconvenience others. Take a few minutes to review your plan to ensure it will do no harm. If you feel any disconnect between your head and your heart, make the necessary adjustments. Remember, you attract the energy you put into the world. You want it to be positive!

7. **Create a wish-list of rewards.** An important part of Bold Freedom is celebrating your success along the way. Think about how you'll reward yourself when you reach your sub-goals and milestones. Will you indulge with a relaxing massage or natural therapy? A date night? A yummy block of organic chocolate? There are so many ways to add to your bank of immunity and make your body feel good. Write down some ideas.

8. **Optional step:** Repeat the process for your business or family. If you'd like to create a plan for your business or family goals, simply repeat the process above. Bold Freedom works for all types of entities. But the most important one is you!

~

Well done for setting your goals. It's not as easy as it sounds! But now you have a clear vision, you can start bringing it to life. In the next section, we'll make your goals even more achievable by designing doable steps. This includes practical tips and examples of how to incorporate Ayurvedic principles and the Bold Freedom method into every day. Have your notebook and calendar handy!

"Authenticity is the daily practice of letting go of who we think we're supposed to be and embracing who we are."

BRENE BROWN

DESIGN DOABLE STEPS

We need a method to create new habits, so we don't default to old ones.

One key to achieving big goals is to enjoy the process. Your headspace needs to be right, so you can reach for the stars feeling happy and healthy. The space you see on your calendar directly relates to your headspace. A clearer calendar equals a clearer mind. It allows you more time to ponder, make decisions, and remain in your personal zone of genius. Think about the most successful people you know. People who excel in their chosen field don't overcrowd their day with "stuff". They outsource, delegate, and get rid of the things they don't really need.

You may not have the luxury of delegating, but you always have room to move. At the very least, you have time to pause. Have you ever noticed the faster you try to get things done, the faster the tasks flood in? Things don't stop until you do. Even in the busiest times, slowing down and taking a breath is the best thing you can do. The aim is to keep your energies balanced, so you're neither pulling or pushing yourself along. Before we move onto the next step – setting practical steps to reach your goals – let's talk about some other ways to balance your energies.

~

One of the most powerful ways is to nourish your body with healthy foods. The food choices you make not only effect how you feel, but how your mind functions. Eating clean, light, nutritious food keeps your gut happy and your mind sharp. It's a win-win situation.

To get the most from your daily meals, focus first on your lunch. In Ayurveda, lunch is prioritised as the largest meal of the day. This is because your digestive ability (called "Agni") is at its peak. As primates, our bile is designed to be optimal when the sun is high, around midday. If a large lunch works for you, you're already off to a great start. But don't despair if it doesn't fit. Everyone is different. Some people do better on two meals a day, around 10am and 4pm. Others might thrive on four small meals a day, without including any snacks. Do what works for you now but try to give more love to your lunch.

Ideally, you want to prepare a hot, satisfying lunch, cooked as freshly as possible. This takes planning and practice – especially if you're used to eating leftovers. While last night's leftovers are quick and convenient, the truth is they are stale. If you can't be home to cook your lunch fresh, prepare it before you leave in the morning. While you're doing your morning prep, you could even pop some chopped veggies in the slow cooker ready for a stew tonight. Suddenly, preparing your lunch in the morning has saved you precious time tonight. Efficiency like this is so empowering!

Another way to give lunch more love (and all your meals, for that matter) is to write out a weekly meal plan. Make a list of meals and ingredients, then schedule shopping and cooking into your week. Avoid doing a big cook-up and freezing meals, because frozen meals are dead food. Yes, the freezer can snap freeze nutrients, but it dulls their life force. Plus, when preparing your food means grabbing a frozen meal, you're not being hands-on and conscious. This makes a world of difference.

As for what to have for lunch, you're only limited by your imagination. How about a one-pot, plant-based wonder with fresh greens on the side? The beauty of one-pot meals is that the food begins to break down as it cooks. This makes the nutrients more readily available. When you consume the food, this beautiful bioavailable goodness can nourish your tissues and give you a natural, long-lasting energy hit.

When you're designing your lunch, aim for a mix of protein, carbs, healthy fats, fibre and trace minerals. An in-season, mostly plant-based diet is a great place to start and will take care of most of your needs. If you're cooking a one-pot wonder, you could include some potatoes in your dish, or add a small serve of rice. However, as a general rule, try to keep your starches low. Too much starch can make you feel heavy – in body and mind. Huge, carb-laden lunches are the main reason why many people suffer from the

"3pm slump". They come crashing down once the quick hit of insulin and energy wears off. We've all been there before!

- **Make a note:** Go back to your weekly template and map out time to prepare your meals. When will you shop for groceries? Can you get to the local farmers market once a week or once a month? In your notebook, jot down a few meal ideas. Start with a one-pot wonder!

If you've never eaten a mostly plant-based diet, don't feel intimidated. There are so many possibilities to delight your palette and make your taste buds dance! In Ayurveda, we keep things simple with the six tastes – sweet, sour, salty, bitter, astringent (think tea and green apple) and pungent (think chilli). The interesting part is trying to include each of these flavours in every meal. If you enjoy cooking, you'll love the balancing act. Unleash your inner Masterchef! If you're new to the kitchen, embrace the challenge. Approach it with a sense of fun. You'll soon see how easy it is to make delicious, healthy lunches in minutes.

Once you've mastered making lunch your main meal, you can start upgrading your other meals. Start by limiting food after dark. One of the worst things you can do for your system is burden it with a heavy dinner and big dessert. If you really can't do without dessert in your day, make it an earlier meal (like afternoon tea), then sip on some soup around 6pm. The other important thing to do is to give yourself time to rest and digest. Allow a few hours break between meals. In old England, they enjoyed a two-hour lunch break – and many countries around the world continue to do this.

~

Good digestive ability, Agni, which is enhanced by eating fresh, seasonal wholefoods, is the key to upgrading how you look and feel. It determines the glow of your skin, the gleam in your eyes, and even how white your teeth are. Then, of course, there's disease prevention. It's no secret that poor quality, processed food is a leading cause of life-threatening diseases. If you don't change what, when and how you eat, you're setting yourself up for disastrous results. It won't be a case of IF you get an autoimmune condition, it will be a case of WHEN. Your body will struggle as best it can for as long as it can, giving you signals along the way. Can you already hear the signals? Are you listening?

If you find yourself feeling lethargic in the mornings, sleepy after lunch, or craving cake at 3pm, it's time to sit up and take notice. These are signs that your body has toxic residue of undigested food – the Ama we referred to earlier. Ama creates congestion in the body and disturbs natural processes. It gets in the way of your energy flow and gives you a fuzzy head. There are many ways you can clear Ama (there's a whole section on that soon), but eating a lighter, early dinner is a great start. Going for a walk after lunch can also help your lymph system eliminate things that aren't serving your body.

- **Make a note:** Write a list of any signals your body has been sending. How could these be related to the foods you're eating? Or when you're eating them? What do you think are the main culprits affecting your health or energy? Notice how your body responds when you swap a large dinner for lunch or stop eating after dark. I bet the results will blow you away!

No matter what your situation, you can fit Ayurveda into your life. The Ayurvedic food principles can be adapted to suit any individual. If you have a specific health concern, talk to your practitioner. You'd be hard pressed to find a practitioner who doesn't endorse a natural, wholefood diet!

~

In addition to changing your diet, changing your inner dialogue is one of the most empowering changes you can make to balance your energies. Do you struggle with procrastination or lack of confidence? Do you give attention to negative thoughts? Take some time to think about why. Get to know yourself better. What makes you angry, sad, afraid or shy? What moves you to swift action? What makes your heart sing? Don't feel limited by what people say you're capable of. Only YOU know your true potential – and only YOU have the power to unlock it. This process takes time as you learn to trust yourself.
Questioning is a great tool for rising above negative self-talk. When a negative thought pops into your head, pause to see if it's actually true. For example, if you hear yourself saying "I don't have the time to meditate right now", try saying "It's not a PRIORITY for me to meditate right now". Which statement really fits? The truth is, you probably do have time to do many things, you just haven't been prioritising them. A simple shift in how you think and what you say can make all the difference.

Another trick that works wonders is re-framing your thoughts and words. Instead of saying "I've GOT to do this", try saying "I GET to do this". Think about how wonderful it is that you GET to move and stretch your body. That you GET to cook yourself a nourishing lunch. That you GET the chance to change your life. Life is a precious gift. It's all about how you see it!

Tip you can try today - Eat that frog!
There will always be something you do in your day that's not your favourite thing. However, you'll probably find when you tackle this first, everything else falls into place. Lean in to the thing you don't love. Make it a priority. Bestselling author Brian Tracy calls this "eating the frog"! You may not enjoy doing it, but just get it done. Then move on with the rest of your day.

~

Now that you have a few tricks up your sleeve to help align your body and mind, let's get back to business. In Step 1, you assessed your current situation. In Step 2, you took stock of your time. In Step 3, you set your goals, including your overarching vision. The next step is to create a plan to bring your goals to life. Don't worry, it's totally doable. Let's start right now, one small step at a time.

STEP 4 SET SMALL STEPS
The overarching goal you set in Step 3 should be a big one. There will be many things that need to happen for you to reach it. Start by picking two or three things to implement this quarter, then break them down into weekly steps. You could start with something small like up-levelling your lunch or re-framing negative thoughts, as we described above. Or start with something totally different. It all depends on your goal and what resonates with you.
To give you an idea of how it works, let's use the example of credit card debt. Say you wanted to clear a credit card debt within a one-year period, what two or three things could you do this quarter to get closer to that goal? Step 1 could be to create a household budget, putting aside $20 a week. Step 2 could be to stop spending on clothes for the next three months. Step 3 could be to cut up your credit card. These are your quarterly steps.

Now break them down further to weekly steps. Using the example above, let's look at Step 1 – creating a household budget and saving $20. Budgeting is a big task. How could you break it down? Maybe you spend the first week assessing your expenditure. The next week you could sit down and write the budget. The following week could be when you begin saving the $20. See how manageable things become when we stop and break them down? Now it's your turn.

1. **Create your quarterly template:** Grab three pieces of paper and plot out the next three months. Write "Week 1", "Week 2", "Week 3" and "Week 4" for each month, using one piece of paper per month. If a month has five weeks, that's a bonus. It means you get more time!

2. **Write your quarterly goals:** At the top of the page, write out the two or three quarterly goals you're going to strive for. These will take you closer to your big yearly goal.

3. **Write your weekly steps:** Now, map out the weekly steps you need to take to reach those monthly goals. You'll be plugging these into your calendar in Step 5, so take some time to get crystal clear on what you want to achieve – and what's possible with your time and resources. You've got a minimum of four weeks every month, sometimes five. That means twelve to fifteen weeks in total. Some weeks may be full, some weeks may be blank. White space is your friend!

When you go through this process, take your time and go into detail. You'll only be doing it once a quarter, so make it really count! If you plan to cut up your credit card, don't just write down "cut up credit card". Write down everything else you'll do around it. How will you celebrate this huge success? Will you have a ceremony? Burn a candle? Reward yourself with a luxurious bath? Treat these wins with the fanfare they deserve. You will have earned it!

~

Tip you can try today - Create triggers
All habits, good and bad, are our response to triggers. Your day is full of tiny triggers that set you in motion for certain behaviours. You might experience conscious triggers, like looking at the clock and knowing it's lunchtime, but triggers are often very subtle. When you're trying to establish a new healthy habit, try aligning it with something you already do. You'll see how much easier it becomes.

For example, I notice I'm more engaged in my afternoon bike ride when I listen to a podcast that's on my to-do list. Yes, it does mean I'm not fully present with the exercise, so I don't do it all the time. But if it makes the difference between doing the bike ride or not, it's worth the compromise. Plus, as well as getting my exercise in, I've listened to the podcast that's been on my list. That's two boxes ticked at once. Just by anchoring these things together. The lesson here is to make things fun for you, whatever that looks like.

If you want to take up a new habit like meditation, anchor it to something you already do. You might try meditating first thing in the morning, as soon as you get out of bed. You're getting out of bed anyway, so set that as your trigger. Have your meditation cushion beside the bed so it becomes easy and automatic.

~

There's a sense of empowerment that comes from taking charge. When you set your own boundaries and parameters, working at a pace that suits you, you'll barely notice change occurring. Before you know it, you'll be ticking off sub-goals and edging towards your big vision. You're already moving in the right direction – creating a space to step into. As you journey into this space, there are no right or wrong decisions. Bold Freedom isn't about being perfect. It's about learning what's best for your unique body and circumstances and doing the best you can. Below is an example of a patient Tim, and his story of Bold Freedom. I hope this inspires you ahead of the next step.

Case Study: Tim
Tim felt stuck in his job. The intense pressure and long hours made him feel tense and miserable, but he couldn't see a way out. His goal was to earn enough money to raise his family and save for retirement. Yet his work was suffering due to poor sleep, and his family didn't see much of him. Even when he was home, Tim was short tempered and snappy. Plus, he was spending about $150 a month on therapies and supplements to feel better. So much for saving money.

It wasn't until Tim paused to look deeply at his habits that he found a way to break the cycle. It was so simple when he broke it down. His first step was to use the Bold Freedom method to organise his work activities. He blocked out his time commitments and started using the resources he had. It took a month to gain traction and start to feel the return. After a month, Tim was more efficient at work. As a result, he was home earlier. He wound down and slept better. Instead of eating out at night, Tim ate dinner at home and took leftovers for lunch the next day. Even though leftovers aren't ideal and making a fresh lunch is preferred, this wasn't possible for Tim at the time. Tim did the best he could, without pressuring himself to be 'perfect'.

The time, energy and money Tim saved in the first thirty days was astounding to him and his family. His health and mood had improved so much, he felt ready to up-level. In the next six months, Tim included walking his dog in his evening routine. He no longer needed to go to the body therapist and was feeling better by himself.

Tim is a perfect example of someone who reversed his trajectory from bleak to brilliant. If Tim had continued with his old habits, he would have used all his money on hospital care, treating his weary body and mind. He would have caused great worry to his family, who were his reason for working all along. Now Tim is living a life he loves. He's happy and healthy – and so are his family. It all started with him!

MAKE TIME FOR ACTION

Trust the process, trust yourself, and show up for the feedback buzz.

How often do you hear or read about the importance of living in the present moment? Being present is brilliant, but you still want to look at the bigger picture. Without a vision and a purpose, you'll find yourself going around in circles. However, when you surrender to a big picture goal, just like you have in the previous chapters, you'll find yourself living more in the present without even needing to try. Yes, your goals will be future-based, but your energy will be directed to the here and now. Your focus is on the small steps and daily moments that take you closer to becoming the person you want to be. This is where the magic happens.

In the previous sections, you established your "why?" and devised a plan for "how?" to reach your goals. The next step is to map the "when?". That's what we'll do in this section. Before we jump right in, let's look at some issues that could pop up.

~

Taking action is the thrilling part, but it can be a stumbling block for some people. Action is where things start to get real. It forces you out of your comfort zone and taking the first steps can be daunting. Your old friends, fear and procrastination, may rear their ugly heads.

No matter how tempting it might seem to stall your plans or compromise, be brave and lean in to your plan. It's a slippery slope back to old thoughts and habits, especially in the first few weeks. When the going gets tough or you feel the fear, return to your "why?" – the reason you wanted to change in the first place. And think about what's REALLY more terrifying – changing or staying the same. Do you really want to struggle on forever with not enough time, not enough energy, not enough money and not enough freedom? Sure, in the short-term things may feel uncomfortable, but keep your eyes on the bigger prize. The new lifestyle you've planned out will bring your body and mind into alignment, creating lasting health and happiness. Isn't that worth some slight discomfort?

Another factor that might pop up is sneaky self-doubt. You've already done the groundwork by setting your goals, determining your vision and creating doable steps. But you might start to worry about your plan. What if you've got it wrong? What if it's too hard? What if you fail? These doubts are common and normal. They are the mind's way of protecting you from failure, but don't let them stop you from getting started! If there's a voice in your head saying, "Why start when I'll probably fail anyway?", use your tools to override it. Changing your inner dialogue, like we described in the previous chapter. Seth Godin pragmatically states, when we say out loud 'it might not work' and we generously and consistently show up to give it a go, that is when we allow our genius the greater voice, over our lizard brain or unrealistic fear.

You may even worry about getting bored. This is also a common response. Remember, our bodies become addicted to stress. They can trick us into thinking stress is enjoyable. However, once you learn to live with ease, you'll realise how much you don't miss stressing! And what's the worst that can happen? You are in control. You'll be reviewing and resetting throughout the journey. There's a review period at the end of each quarter, where you can pivot and tweak your plans. You won't want to deviate to much from your vision, but there's plenty of room to play around. Just start and see how you go!

A final worry that may arise is how people will respond to your new lifestyle. What will your family and friends think? How will your actions impact them? Will they support you? What if you can't accommodate their needs like you've done in the past? If you're used to prioritising others' needs, this can be a tricky one. But remember to fill your own cup first. When you are happy, healthy and feeling your best, this will radiate throughout your life. Whatever roles you perform – parent, worker, business owner etc – you'll perform at a higher level. And when emergencies or circumstances arise, you'll respond to them with poise and grace. One thing at a time. Don't let the fear of what "might" happen stop you from starting your own journey. Once you're plans are in motion, I bet you'll be pleasantly surprised by how others' respond. People will have your back!

- **Make a note:** Write down any worries or fears you have about beginning to journey to Bold Freedom. Just the simple act of getting them down on paper will be powerful and liberating. Once you have them written down, challenge them. Play Devil's Advocate. Is there a genuine reason to be afraid or is it simply your fear response kicking in, protecting you against the threat of failure?

While you're there, start thinking of ways you can combat these fears – and other potential pitfalls – when they inevitably pop up along the way. Create a contingency plan with practical solutions. For example, if you're unable to prepare your lunch in the morning, what healthy options are available close to the office? If you sleep in and miss your exercise routine, how else could you incorporate movement into your day? When it comes to success, there's no such thing as being over-prepared! Write down your ideas now so you can come back to them when you need to.

~

Bold Freedom is intended to help you overcome your inner struggles and poise you for the grace of health. It honours the natural design of your body. However, if your body has been unaligned for a long time, it could take a while to feel the benefits. Try not to get caught up in the tiny details when things get tough. Keep your mind on your yearly goal, follow the steps you have set out, and surrender completely to the process. The more feedback you get from your body, the more you'll learn to trust yourself. You'll realise your body knows best. You'll begin to nurture that ability to decide for yourself, to make healthy choices, and to realise everything can be figured out one way or another. As Marie Forleo puts it, 'everything's figureoutable!'. You'll identify when you need more sleep, what foods make your body feel alive, and what activities make your heart sing.

To give you some practical examples of how other Bold Freedom followers have overcome fear, doubt and other challenges, here are some case studies. These stories show how easy it is to make Bold Freedom work for you. They also show you how the planets align when you tap in to your intuition.

Case Study: Sarah
Sarah thought she wanted more money to feel healthy and happy. Her vision was to earn enough to look after her young family – to comfortably pay for expenses with ease. Sarah set an annual goal to make more money through her market stall business. She actioned this goal for a quarter, investing all her time and energy into her market stall. However, at the end of the quarter she realised this plan wasn't working. Sarah was making more money, but her family relationships were suffering. She began resenting her time at the stall. There was a misalignment in her goal to make money and her desire to provide for her family. Sarah decided to change direction. She kept her goal to provide for the household but focused her energies more inward. She took a step back from the market stall, treating it more like a hobby business. Without the demands of full-time work, Sarah had more time to provide for her family. She cooked nourishing meals and spent more time helping her children with homework. Around the same time, Sarah's husband got a promotion. The money started flowing in. It wasn't the path Sarah expected to take, but the destination was the same. Health, happiness and money began flowing as soon as Sarah was true to her desires. Her market stall business is still running, but now she enjoys her time there instead of seeing it as a burden.

Case Study: Judy
Judy suffered from a chronic cough. She'd always called herself "a cougher". This was part of her vocabulary. Judy's goal was to rid herself of the pesky cough that was impacting her life. She snored heavily, making her wake up grumpy – and she kept her husband up all night. Herbal tonics relieved her symptoms, but only temporarily. As Judy journeyed through Bold Freedom, she looked deeply at her thoughts and desires. She realised she was looking after others, never thinking of her herself. There was no flow in her life. The element of water was sorely lacking. Judy began following an Ayurvedic recommendation to start sipping hot water throughout the day, sometimes adding lemon and ginger. Instead of calling herself a "cougher", Judy became

"a hydrator". She began paying more attention to her food, noticing how cold foods like ice-cream triggered her cough. She also started taking time for herself, making space to read a book or go for a walk. Within weeks she stopped coughing and snoring. Her doctor and husband were amazed – and Judy had never felt better. Judy's story shows that treating a symptom in isolation doesn't treat the real problem. All Judy needed to cure her cough was to get flow back into her life. She achieved this by tapping into her intuition, nourishing her body with lots of warm, loving water and making space for self-care.

~

Let's schedule time for your own action. We'll do this by populating your calendar with your quarterly actions and weekly steps. Think of your calendared plan like a piece of music. It brings rhythm to your day, your week, your year. It's not a thing that binds you, it's a platform that allows new opportunities to arise. Bold Freedom is about writing your own song – your own Ayur Veda. You can add layers, turn the volume up and down, and pause to reflect. Just keep tuning in.

I highly recommend you switch to a digital calendar at this point, as there will be quite a lot of detail to fill in. I like a digital calendar because you can easily move things around or use colours to code tasks. But if you prefer paper, that's perfectly fine. Do what works for you!

STEP 5 SCHEDULE YOUR TIME

1. **Set a start date.** Make a commitment to begin on the next Monday from today, regardless of what month you're in. It takes a few days to nestle into the Bold Freedom method. By giving yourself space to set things up and look at your plan for a few days, you'll be warmed up when next Monday comes. You'll be ready to step into your week with clarity and confidence. Mark the day in your calendar now.

2. **Realign to time.** In a perfect world, you'd start your journey on January 1. However, as we've established so far, Bold Freedom isn't about being perfect. You can start your journey at any time in any of the four quarters. The journey will end in the calendar year, but you can carry over your annual goal. Everything will balance out. For now, simply determine

how much time you have left in the current calendar year. How many weeks left in this quarter? These are the weeks you'll start filling in.

3. **Schedule your strategic block.** One day a week (preferably on the same day so it becomes habit), block out two to three hours around your other commitments – the one's you mapped out in Step 2. This is your strategic block. You'll use this time to implement the weekly steps you set in Step 4. If possible, schedule your strategic block in the morning before daily distractions takeover. If you can only do an evening or weekend, I recommend the weekend as it's more aligned to your circadian rhythms. Your mind wants to wind down in the evenings, not fire up for action!

4. **Make time for fun.** Now, give yourself a blank day (or at least half a day) purely for fun. This is your time to do anything you like. Scheduling this time is so freeing and it will make your journey much more enjoyable. Trust that you'll reach your goals because you've dedicated time to them. You still have plenty of time for fun!

5. **Check for white space.** Now you have your essential commitments, strategic block and fun built in, check that your calendar has white space. White space allows you to shift things around and respond to changes in your plans. It's a contingency for when things pop up – like a family emergency or a special event. White space gives you the time to smoothly switch gear from one task or area in your life to another.

~

Congratulations on making the time! See how simple it can be to find the time to live well? Have you ever heard the saying "time expands to meet the task at hand"? If you have all day to do a task, chances are you'll take all day! If you have space, you'll fill it. If you have money, you'll spend it. This is human nature. By making time to meet your goals, half the work is already done. You have made the commitment. All you need to do now is show up. Make the changes you promised to make. Your body and mind will give you feedback along the way that will help keep the momentum going. Why not try it right now? Here's a mini exercise to warm you up for the next section.

Make a note: What can you do in the next hour that your body will love you for? It could be as simple as making a cup of herbal tea, stretching your body, or going outdoors. Write your idea down now, along with the time you'll do it in the next hour. When that time comes, stop reading and do it. Notice how your body responds and rewards you for showing up.

TWO: RESET THE SCENE

MOVE THE FURNITURE

The space we create outside our body impacts what happens inside our body.

The previous chapter of Bold Freedom was about organising your time. This chapter is all about organising your space. The goal is to create an environment that sets you up for success and makes you feel happy, aligned and calm. It's about reducing the clutter in your life and creating a haven to truly thrive in. Only when you feel calm in your external space can wonderful change occur inside.

Space takes many forms. It can refer to your physical space, your headspace and even white space on your calendar. When we talk about space in this section, we're referring mostly to your physical environment – the places you live, work, rest and play. When you feel at ease in your physical space, you can slash your stress significantly. This creates a stable foundation from which health can grow. Think about it. Have you ever noticed how it's much easier to work at a clean desk or relax in a tidy house? Space has a profound effect on your thoughts, moods and actions. When you can move around your environment freely, knowing everything is in its place, you flow through life with ease and grace. On the other hand, when there's chaos in your environment there's often chaos in your mind. Too much "stuff" gets in the way.

Think about the many efforts you've made to get healthy in the past. Is it possible these were short lived because your stuff got in the way? Could you have created a chaotic environment by burdening your space with too many things? Maybe you invested in a fancy piece of exercise equipment, packed your pantry with superfoods, or shopped up a storm for the latest yoga wear. Your intentions may have been good, so why didn't they translate to results? The truth is, all the stuff in the world won't work without goals and triggers.

When it comes to creating healthy habits, your gear is less important than time and space. Let's use the yoga wear as an example. Say you buy a new yoga outfit with the good intention of practicing yoga. The outfit looks great in the shop and you feel excited to get started. You even put the outfit on when you get home. However, you never get around to doing the yoga. Why? Well, you made the effort to invest in the gear, but did you organise your time and space? Did you set a time to practice? Did you decide where you would practice – a local studio, at home, in the park? These decisions set the scene for action. Without making time and space, it's unlikely you'll take action. Your gorgeous new yoga outfit will end up in the back of a drawer – just another thing taking up space.

Now think about how you could change this scenario. How could you make it easier to achieve your goal of practising yoga? What steps could you take? Say you decide to practise at home in the morning, that's the time and the place taken care of. Now what resources do you need? Do you really need that yoga gear now, or could you practice in your PJs? Would your money be better spent on a yoga mat, rather than an expensive pair of leggings no one will see? With your time, place and gear sorted, you can go further into setting the scene. Lay out your yoga mat in the living room or a quiet place in your home. That way it's ready, waiting every morning. You might even make this space more enticing by adding a salt lamp or some crystals. Whatever makes you feel at ease. Finally, think about how you could link morning yoga to an existing trigger to create a habit, like we discussed in the previous chapter. What's the first thing you do when you get out of bed? If you drink a large glass of water, link your yoga habit to that. As soon as you finish your water, that's your cue to hit the mat. Give it a few weeks and you'll see it becomes automatic! Once you develop the yoga habit THEN reward yourself with that new outfit. You'll enjoy it so much more!

Make a note: Think about a time when you've prioritised gear over time and space. Maybe you have a drawer of amazing yoga outfits or an exercise machine collecting dust. Perhaps you have an expensive blender but you're yet to make a single smoothie. Write down as many examples as you can, including the missing links between intention and action. This list will come in very handy as you progress through this chapter. Hint: You're going to use it or lose it!

~

Now you understand the importance of space, let's look closely at your environment. Visualise the physical spaces you spend the most time in, starting with your home. Walk through your home in your mind and picture what each room looks like. How much stuff do you really use and how much is just filling up space? You'll probably notice the big things first, like furniture and appliances. But don't forget about the smaller items. What's in your bathroom cupboard or that notorious bottom drawer? How crowded is your wardrobe? Your bookshelf? Your garage?

The things in your space define you, so think about what they all mean. Have you chosen them personally or somehow just ended up with them? How do your things make you feel? Happy, irritated, indifferent? Most of all, think about how PRACTICAL your things are. Do you use that chair? Do those clothes still fit? Is that cereal out of date? I bet you'll be surprised by the number of things you don't use or need. Freeing yourself from these material possessions is such an empowering thing to do. Not only does it create space in your physical environment, it creates space in your mind. Plus, you'll make room for new things and experiences. Things that you have specifically chosen, that align to your values and bring joy to your life.

Let me share a personal example. I recently got rid of two couches that were taking up space in my living room. They were beautiful couches and it wasn't easy to part with them. However, I realised they were in the way and I'd been keeping them "just in case". Just in case a huge crowd of visitors popped in. When I stopped to think about it, I realised this was an unlikely scenario. Even without the couches, I'd have ample room to accommodate four of five visitors. How often would I need more seats than that? Even if I did host a party, couldn't I figure something out? Most people stand around talking anyway!

Now that the couches are gone, I have an inviting, open floor space to move my body. I use this space to jump on my rebounder and do my yoga practice. I also have a similar space in my bedroom, just for sitting and meditation. Some people have said to me, "please don't get rid of any more furniture!", but the space I've created is pleasing to me. I love having a room I can move around in. It makes me feel free. Plus, it's much more practical. I look forward to doing my daily rebounder session because the space I've created makes it easy. If I had to fight with furniture and feel enclosed in a crowded room, it wouldn't be as appealing.

Another benefit of having this dedicated space is that it keeps my goals front of mind. Every time I see the space in the living room, I'm reminded that staying fit is one of my goals. I don't even need to have the rebounder out! Let's consider another example to illustrate what I mean. I know many who put exercise equipment in their garage, so it doesn't clutter their living space. You might think this would create an "out of sight, out of mind" scenario, but not if you anchor it to an existing habit. Say you come in through the garage every afternoon. This could be your trigger. When you see the equipment, you're reminded of your goal to be free of back pain, get stronger or lose weight. This is your signal to get changed and get that exercise done. Imagine how you'd feel if you passed the equipment every day and didn't show up to exercise? My guess is not great! A subtle cue, like seeing the equipment, is all it takes to create change. You can create these cues in your environment any way that works for you.

Make a note: Write down one small change you could make in your home to set the scene for success. How could you link a healthy habit to an existing trigger? Could you leave your lunchbox on the bench overnight to prompt you to prepare lunch in the morning? Leave a bottle of water beside your bed to drink as soon as you wake up? Once you see how easy it is, you will likely think of many changes. You don't need to stop at one!

~

STEP 6 SET THE SCENE

You've now got a sense of your physical space and how to align it with your plan. The next step is to follow through with some spring cleaning! This is a process you'll do every quarter, regardless of the season. The aim is to create an environment that's in sync with your vision, that makes you feel at ease, and that's functional. If there are things in your space that make you feel stuck or irritated, now's the time to say goodbye. Not great at goodbyes? Be brave and lean in. Many people struggle with letting go, but I promise you'll feel like a weight's been lifted. Here are some tips to help you through.

- **Set dedicated time for spring cleaning.** Grab your calendar and block out time for a spring clean every quarter. You might block out a full day, half day, or a couple of hours each week for a few weeks. It all depends on what you prefer, how much clutter you have, and the time you have available. Do what works for you. Just make sure you block it out.

- **Tackle a small space first.** When the time comes, start with a small space. It could be a single cupboard, drawer, or corner of a room. Clear one space at a time and build up to a whole room. Then move to the next room, and so on, until you've completed the whole house.

- **Consider starting with your clothes.** One of the easiest places for some people to start is their wardrobe. Go through your wardrobe, piece by piece, and work out what still serves you. As Marie Kondo wonderfully poses the question, does your clothing spark joy? Does it fit? Do you still like it? If not, could you alter it or turn it into something else? If the answer is no, let it go. You could donate your unwanted clothes to charity, give them to a friend, or simply get rid of them.

- **Do away with unwanted decorations.** The next thing I recommend you tackle are ornaments and decorative items. Look at each one and decide how it makes you feel. Does it look beautiful, or add colour or texture? Does it make you feel good? Would it look better somewhere else? If not, why keep it? This simple act of stocktaking can feel so good. Even if you just lift things up, clean underneath them, then put them back down.

- **Don't fear the furniture.** Moving large items like furniture out of your home can feel radical, especially if you've been raised to collect things – to desire a house with two couches, four chairs, one kitchen table. Please don't be afraid. Go back to the simple principles you used with your clothes and ornaments. Does the furniture serve you? Does it make you feel delighted? Is it practical? The size of the item is irrelevant. How it makes you feel and function is what really matters.

- **Think outside the box.** Be curious and creative. If you're on the fence about a certain item, think about ways you could transform it. Could you repurpose it into something else? I remember buying a beautiful kitchen table, chopping the legs off, and turning it into a coffee table. It was a bold thing to do, which shocked a few visitors, but it was perfect for me. I had two young children at the time, who spent hours playing on the floor. The stumpy-legged table was incredibly practical. Plus, I thought it looked great!

- **Consider other people.** When you spring clean your home, consider the people who share your space. Think about how your decisions will impact them. Chop the legs of your table if you want, but only if it doesn't inconvenience others. In my example above, the kids loved the makeshift coffee table. It benefited everyone in the house. However, if I had thrown out all their noisy toys (even if they irritated me) that would have been a different story. Be kind, be practical and involve others. As you repeat this process each quarter, the family will fall into natural alignment.

- **Be honest and ruthless.** If you don't like it, don't need it, and you can't reuse it, don't be afraid to be ruthless. You know that exercise where you imagine that your house is on fire and you have minutes to grab your most prized possessions? Think about it like that. What would you run through fire for and what would you happily leave behind? There's no wrong or right answers. In fact, the things that you value most might seem completely illogical to other people. I have a perfect example. I lived overseas with young children for many years and we put most of our belongings in storage. However, I did take my favourite wok, because preparing my food is important to me. I also took almost everything from the kids' bedrooms – their books, toys, and favourite blankets. I wanted to ensure that, wherever we went, things would feel comfortable and familiar. Some people thought I was crazy, but this was important to me. It allowed me to create a space that was perfectly aligned with my values, even on the other side of the world.

- **Seek a second opinion:** If you really struggle with spring cleaning, get support from a friend. A good friend will make the process fun and won't be afraid to ask twice, "Do you REALLY want to keep that?" A good idea is to create a pile of "maybe" items. If you're stuck on a certain item, put it in the "maybe" pile. Then grab a friend to help you decide. They may even take some things off your hands!

~

How light do you feel just thinking about spring cleaning and blocking out your time? When you complete this process, you'll see how your foggy head clears as you clear the space around you. This quarterly practice of aligning your space with care and thought will serve you well throughout Bold Freedom. Plus, once your space is decluttered, you'll find it so much easier to maintain. In fact, if you make small daily efforts to keep things in their place, the quarterly clean will be a breeze. You may only need to do one or two rooms each quarter. And you'll drastically reduce your time. Challenge yourself to make each quarter as quick and streamlined as possible by maintaining your space in between cleans.

RELATIONSHIP REVIEW

We crave connection with ourselves and others. Make your connections matter.

Your Bold Freedom journey is personal and individual, but you don't journey through life alone. Your partner, family, friends and colleagues all influence you to some extent. Just as you influence them. The relationships you have with other people can bring infinite joy and happiness to life. Human connections are a beautiful thing! However, they can also be harmful if you don't surround yourself with the right people. In this section, we'll explore the key relationships in your life and how to optimise them. You'll learn how to align your relationships to your goals and create harmony in your inner circle. You'll also learn to recognise when relationships aren't serving you, including what you can do to remedy this.

~

When people truly love and value you, they have your best interests at heart. They care about your health and happiness and they want you to be well. You want the same for them. Relationships with these people are fluid and easy. They give you energy, rather than take it. When you're around these people, you can be honest about your goals, aims and purpose, because you know they'll have your back – even if they think you're being strange, different or completely crazy. At the end of the day, if your goals make you happier and healthier, your loved ones will get on board.

Think about your closest relationships and how they influence your health and happiness. Do the people around you bring out your best qualities?

Do you bring out theirs? Do you love, respect and support each other? In the first chapter we talked about successful people and how they surround themselves with like-minded souls. No matter what type of success you're striving for, this notion holds true. Human behaviour rubs off and habits are extremely contagious. In fact, studies have shown that we become the average of the five people we spend the most time with. So, if you want to be a healthy person, hang around healthy people. If you want to be a happy person, hang around happy people. However, if you want to be someone who's tired, stressed and miserable, spend time with miserable people. I guarantee their energy will rub off!

Make a note: Write down the five people you spend the most time with, excluding small children. Think of your partner, family, friends and colleagues. How healthy is the company you keep? What are the positive traits of your loved ones and how do they influence you? Do they have any unhealthy habits? Have you picked these up? You could even go one step further and look at the five people around your five people. Even they have an indirect impact on your life. Write everything down in as much detail as you can. You might find things you've never noticed before. Bold Freedom is full of surprises!

~

We spoke at the beginning of this book about filling your own cup first. Prioritising your needs is vitally important. However, when you surround yourself with the right people, it's natural to want to care for them. You'll do a much better job if you are healthy, happy and well. When you recognise and honour your own truth, you create a wonderful ripple effect. You become more in tune with others around you – their needs and their desires. It's almost like a super power. On the other hand, if you're coming from a place of depleted energy, you're no good to anyone. This doesn't just apply to your family. It applies to work, sport, or in any sort of team environment. You need energy to give energy! So how do you generate this energy? It starts with self-care. So next time you feel selfish for taking your full lunch break or meditating for ten minutes away from the kids, ask yourself who'd really suffer if you neglected these acts of self-care.

By being kind to yourself, you're being kind to others. If there are people in your life who don't recognise this, think about why that might be. It could be that they are self-centred or rude. But it could also be because you have unknowingly created a culture where your needs are perceived as secondary. This is quite a common scenario. When you're over-reactive to other people and prioritise their needs over your own, you create an expectation. People expect you to always be there. When they say "jump!" you say, "how high?". Does that sound familiar? If this rings true – with your kids, boss, partner or friends – try not to feel resentful. Your loved ones are probably unaware they are making you feel this way. Instead of feeling upset, think about how your actions may have contributed and how you can change the situation. How can you empower yourself and reset expectations? You'll learn some tricks in the following step.

~

STEP 7 ALIGN YOUR RELATIONSHIPS

- **Revisit your calendar.** Before you can positively influence others, you want to be clear on your own priorities. Set aside half an hour each day this week to reflect on the calendar you have created. Reinforce your vision and goals, including your big "why?". This may seem like wasted time but trust the investment will pay off threefold. You'll stay stronger in the face of challenges (like demanding colleagues and pushy friends) and so many opportunities for relief will arise.

- **Get your family involved.** The people around you will be a source of support throughout your Bold Freedom journey. Now's time to involve your household – as much or as little as you like. You could create a family calendar with specific family goals, or simply share your goals with them. Let them know what you're doing and lead by example. Invite them to help you create the weekly meal plan, go grocery shopping, or enjoy a family walk after dinner. If your family are hesitant at first, don't despair. It can take time (up to a year in some cases) but eventually you'll notice collective shifts. Remember, 40% of what you do is habit and you share those habits with your household. Your positive habits will rub off. All in good time.

- **Don't forget the kids.** If you have small children, include them as much as possible. No matter how young they are, it's never too early to start good habits. Kids love to feel included and, by involving them in your plans, you're setting them up for health and happiness.

- **Communicate on team decisions:** When making decisions about your shared space, a little conversation goes a long way. Say you want to move the couch to create more exercise room. When you raise this with your family, there are tactics you can use. First, pick your time and ask permission. You might say, "I'd like to talk about the furniture, is now a good time?" Or, "I'd like to talk about the furniture, when's a good time for you?". Once you're in the conversation, be clear on the reasons behind your proposal. Why does moving the couch matter? Think of this almost like a sales pitch. Sell the benefits to your family. For example, you could say. "When I exercise I feel so much happier and having this space would mean so much. I know it's easier for you when I'm happy, so I think this is a good move". There's a bonus tip on communicating later in this chapter.

- **Be open to input.** When you raise ideas with your family, be willing to listen to their concerns. Give your family some "buy in" so they feel part of the decision. If you explain your reasoning clearly, your family are likely to get on board. Plus, as a bonus, they'll be more likely to hold you accountable. Expect to hear something like, "Hey, I noticed you haven't exercised this week, even though we moved the couch. Does that mean we can put the couch back? Are you going to exercise or not?". This type of input is fantastic as it keeps you focused on your goals and unites the family unit. Your victories will become their victories. What a wonderful thought!

- **Prepare to compromise.** Remember things don't need to be perfect. The personal calendar you created is based on an ideal scenario, but sometimes you will need to compromise. For example, you may want to sit down for a family dinner by 6pm. This is a perfect time to eat because your bile is still active until the sun goes down. However, if other members of your household don't get home until 7pm this is simply not possible. In this example you have two options. You could wait until 7pm and eat together. Or you could eat first at 6pm then join your family later as a table companion. You could even change tactics each quarter and see what works for you. You may find you prefer to eat at 7pm after all – that the emotional benefits of eating as a family outweigh the physical benefits of eating earlier.

- **Set personal boundaries:** Involving your family will help you create harmony and alignment in your environment, but you're still entitled to some personal space. If you know you need an hour to yourself each morning, let your family know. Just like group decisions, if you explain why this time is so important, your loved ones will respect your wishes. It all comes back to communication.

- **Ask for support.** As humans, we are so often reluctant to ask for support. We assume our loved ones should know what we need, but we can't expect them to read minds! Reaching out for support from your family not only helps you navigate issues, it encourages teamwork and communication. For example, if you're feeling a bit lost or down, you could say to a family member, "I'm not feeling great, but I don't know why. Will you help me work it out?". Figure things out together. This is how you grow together.

- **Cut ties when you need to.** Unfortunately, there are times when certain relationships simply don't serve you. If someone in your life is taking more energy than they give, or hurting or disrespecting you, it's OK to end that relationship. I've personally ended spousal and community relationships before. These decisions were difficult at the time, but essential to maintain my integrity – plus wellness for myself and my children. If you find yourself in an unhealthy relationship and you can't find a way to solve the issues, be brave and walk away. Recognise the relationship has served its purposes and honour your own spirit.

~

I hope you can see how resetting the scene of your life will support you during your journey to good health. On the surface, the benefits of these changes may seem emotional and external, but trust the internal changes are just as profound. When you ditch the things that no longer serve you, allowing yourself to feel nurtured and supported, your body responds to its very core. Surrounding yourself with the things and people you love is what enables your body to naturally detox. When you feel supported, so does your body. Your body tissues can relax and let go, releasing any Ama or tension you've been storing. When your body and mind are at ease, you'll feel aligned from the inside out. The scene will be set for wonderful things! To show you how this works in action, here's a case study and a quick tip you can try today.

Case study: Amy
Amy was getting up at 4:30am to practice self-care before her young family awoke. If she had any leftover time, she used it to complete household duties and to work on her small business. On the surface, Amy was doing everything right. She was making time for self-care and being productive. Yet she was still feeling tired and out of sorts. When Amy applied the Bold Freedom method, two things came to light. Amy realised she was not nurturing her relationship with her husband. Instead of spending time with him at night, she was going to sleep with the kids so that she could wake up early. Amy also realised she was out of sync with her own body rhythm. She was going to bed too early. Once Amy noticed these things, she tweaked her routine slightly. She began spending half an hour of quality time with her husband each night. She went to bed a little later and began waking at 5am. The changes to Amy's household were striking. Just by shifting things half an hour, Amy was able to connect with her husband. This allowed her to identify and communicate where she craved support in all areas of life. Her husband stepped up to provide this support, feeling more loved and valued himself. Plus, the kids benefited from having two happy parents, who were no longer tired or disconnected. The energy in the whole household changed for the better.

Tip you can try today - Tailor your language to suit your audience.
A great communication tip I learned from relationship coach, Matthew Hussey, is to tailor your language to suit your audience – specifically males and females. This can be particularly helpful when you're talking to your partner or family about making a change within the household. Matthew found that males often respond more positively when you phrase your question in a way that considers their feelings. For example, "Would you mind helping me with the dishes?" or "Would you mind helping me moving the couch?". On the other hand, females tend to respond more favourably when you ask in a way that makes them feel helpful. For example, "Can you help me do the dishes?" or "Can you help me figure this out?". This trick won't work for everyone. We are all unique and delightfully different, but I found it very interesting. Try it and see how you go. Think of it as a fun experiment!

THREE: KNOW HOW YOUR BODY WORKS

CLEAR ANY BLOCKS
Change can only happen in space.

Congratulations on your journey so far. In the previous chapters, you created much needed time and space, setting the scene for health to bloom. You're already off to a flying start! Now it's time to get down to business by learning how your body works. In this chapter, we'll explore the wonderful complexities of the human body, including how you can apply Ayurvedic principles to help your body feel its best. There's a lot of information to cover, so we'll tackle it in two steps. The first step is to clear any blocks and reduce Ama.

In Ayurveda, we use the term Ama to describe anything that blocks and congests us. Ama can take many forms – from the thoughts we have, to the energy we breathe, to the fuel we absorb, and even what we watch on TV. Ama can be physical or emotional. It can be generated by diet, movements, relationship and beliefs. Ama comes and goes naturally over the course of a day. If our digestive capacity (Agni) is functionally well, it prevents the toxic residue of undigested substances from being stored in our bodies. However, if Agni is not optimised, Ama builds up. Toxic Ama is our greatest limitation to enjoying life. It corrupts the messages between body and mind, causing cravings for substances that don't serve us. It's what stops us from honouring our truth and fulfilling our deepest heart's desires – which is exactly what you're here to do.

Clearing Ama by improving Agni – digestive capacity – is one of the most critical parts of your Bold Freedom journey. It's also one of the most challenging. However, trust that when you clear your blocks, you pave the way for transformation. See this challenge as a gift. This is your opportunity to step up, take charge and overcome your greatest obstacles. It's your chance to finally break free of anything that has held you back. You may have to face some demons and even confront some home truths – but you WILL reap rewards on the other side. Be brave and trust the process. This is where the magic happens!

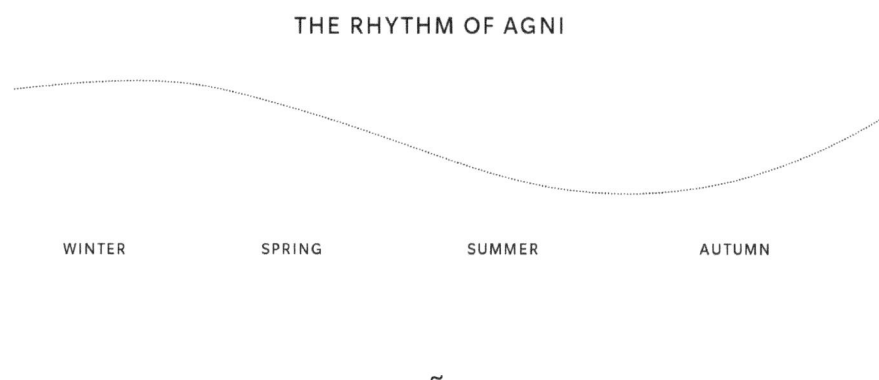

~

STEP 8 CLEAR AMA
When it comes to clearing blocks in your life, it helps to understand the difference between physical and emotional blocks. Physical blocks are usually more obvious, so let's start there. An example of a physical block could be something as simple as a scheduling conflict. For example, say you need to take the kids to soccer training at 4pm. However, 4pm is your body's preferred time to go for a brisk walk outside and have a stretch. The time factor is actually a physical block to honouring your body's desires. Physical blocks can also be related to your body's physiology, like belly fat making it difficult to bend or causing discomfort during exercise.

In the past, you may have used these blocks as an excuse to avoid doing exercise. Change can be scary, and the mind welcomes any excuse to avoid doing "the thing" we're afraid of. This is completely normal – but it can stop now. It takes confidence and courage to confront what's REALLY happening, but you absolutely can do it. The truth is, physical blocks can usually be overcome with relative ease. Go for a walk in the park when you do the soccer drop-off – and persevere with those bending exercises. The more you bend, the easier it will become as your metabolism increases, you feel less stressed, and the belly fat begins to melt away.

Ayurvedic remedies often bring a "win-win" solution, clearing Ama and improving Agni at the same time. It's true that finding the solution may take some extra effort, but you are worth that effort. You and your kind hearted big vision for a thriving life deserve to go that extra mile! Plus, when you look at challenges in terms of your big picture purpose, you're already half way there. Often all you need is some time to ponder. Give yourself time to do the work. Consider where you do your best thinking. Is it in the shower, on the train, or anytime you're present in your own body? Simply spending your lunch break outdoors, away from your phone, can be a great way to recharge and reflect. When you give yourself time and space, you'll find that most physical blocks can be overcome.

Make a note: An effective way to identify physical blocks is to look back at your calendar.
Does anything new stand out? Can you identify any conflicts? Write down any physical blocks or barriers that could stop you from reaching your goals. Then write down your solutions. How could you reshuffle your time to better align with your goals? Could you ask your husband to drop the kids at soccer? Could you hire a trainer to help you with exercise and make those bending movements easier? Being proactive with blocks is one of the best ways to overcome them.

~

Now that we've covered physical blocks, let's explore emotional blocks. When a block is emotional, the solution isn't always as simple as rearranging your schedule. Emotional blocks are deep-seated and can arise from experiences long past. They could stem from moments in childhood you can't remember, or from DNA passed down by your ancestors. They could also arise from recent traumas, self-limiting beliefs, or negative energies you have absorbed from people and experiences over the years. There really is no limit to what they could be.

The problem with emotional blocks is that they can permeate your thoughts and actions without you even noticing. They can be all-encompassing, shaping every aspect of your life – work, relationships, your approach to health. You see, Ama isn't just a block, it's also a corrupter. Emotions are feelings that have become affected by previous experiences. They arise from the stories we tell ourselves, often over many years. If you can't determine the feeling behind a negative emotion, you can't make sense of it in your environment. This means you can't let it go and the emotion lingers in your body. When negative emotions aren't dissolved they are stored as Ama, often in fat cells. Good Agni helps clear Ama overnight – and you can help things along with seasonal detoxes and lifestyle changes. However, when emotional blocks aren't cleared, they tend to manifest in physical symptoms. This makes them even more toxic. Let me give you an example.

The most common diseases in our modern society are autoimmune conditions or diseases of congestion. Physically, these arise from poor lifestyle habits, like eating poorly, not exercising or not breathing deeply. The evidence on this is clear. But let's look beyond the surface for a moment. What emotional blocks cause people to make these poor lifestyle choices? What causes someone to repeatedly overeat unhealthy food, even though it makes them feel bad? What makes someone shy away from moving their body, despite receiving doctor's orders? Do you see what I'm getting at here?

In cases like this, there MUST be an underlying emotional cause because everything we need to live healthy lives is at our disposal! Think about the incredible opportunities we have today compared to our ancestors. We have access to an abundance of fresh, nutritious foods. We can choose from an array of amazing exercise options. We have transport, technology and instant access to millions of resources around the world. So why are we still struggling? On paper, it should be so easy to stay happy and healthy. But emotional blocks aren't black and white. They're complex, layered and incredibly personal. They take time to unravel.

If you feel like you're doing all the right things, yet you don't feel healthy or fulfilled, you could have an emotional block. Perhaps you're prone to self-sabotage because you don't think you're worth the effort. Maybe you have a fear of failure because you grew up trying to please your parents. Anything is possible. If you've been struggling for many years, you may never have taken the time to consider what's blocking you. When you're frazzled, desperate or driven by fear, your mind doesn't think clearly. Plus, if you have no memory of the events that shaped you – if they stem from early childhood or were passed down through your DNA – of course you feel confused!
To make matters more complex, emotional blocks are like double-edged swords. In addition to the primary problem – the emotional block itself – it can be stressful to feel like you're "doing the work" but not seeing the results. When this happens, it creates a cycle of stress in the body and can

have a negative impact on self-trust. There's not a superfood or supplement on the planet that can rectify this alone. Even if your nutrition is on point, your body will be using all the nutrients to manage stress and prevent mineral loss – not to nourish and heal your body. The best relief you can give yourself is to take time out and break the cycle. Focus on relieving stress as your number one priority. Have you ever noticed how a happy person eating a hamburger can seem healthier than a stressed vegan? You can't underestimate the impact of stress. Clearing it is a great starting point.

The aim of this chapter is to help you consider, identify and clear blocks, so you can move unobstructed towards your goals. Patience, perseverance and compassion are essential as you navigate these waters. Please treat yourself with kindness. Let's start with a simple journaling exercise.

Make a note: Think about your past experiences related to your wellness journey. What emotional obstacles have stood in your way? Can you pinpoint any feelings, thoughts or moments that have stopped you from reaching your goals? If you identify any emotional blocks – like a limiting self-belief or poor self-esteem – write them down. If you feel stuck, that's OK too. Simply write down how you feel, just like a stream of consciousness. Just be tapping into your emotions and writing down what comes up, you're already starting to clear your blocks.

~

No matter what your journaling brought up, I commend you for your bravery. Facing your emotions can be can be painful, ugly and embarrassing – even when you're the only one in the room. Wherever you're at right now, accept yourself without judgement. It's very easy to get caught in the cycle of overanalysing and asking, "How did I get here?". Please don't be hard on yourself. Understand that sometimes your pain needs to reach a peak before you feel strong enough to act. Sometimes the fear of staying the same must become worse than the fear of changing. If you have reached this tipping point, see it as a good thing. When you break down you can break through. And when you break through, the possibilities are endless. When each of your cells can communicate and move freely, without being shackled by blocks, your body's natural intelligence kicks in. Your body will start using stored nutrients and resources to full effect. Your head will become clear and you can begin to heal. Naturally, effortlessly, from the inside out.

That's what we're aiming for here.

Keep this vision in your mind as you journey through Bold Freedom, especially when things feel tough. This program works as hard as you do. Trust that your work will lead to results. Invest the time. Remember, you are worth it!

~

Now that you understand the difference between physical and emotional blocks, and you've started tuning into your deepest self, let's look at some other ways to clear Ama. There are many Ayurvedic practices you can use to support your body through the healing process. The good news is, you can start today.

In Ayurveda we follow a daily routine, which we call "Dinacharya". We'll be delving deep into Dinacharya in the next section, but I wanted to share some of the key principles you can follow to help you detox every day. Think of these tips as an appetiser for the main course that's to follow. We've touched on some of these before and we'll continue to come back to them. There's a whole world to explore!

- **Eat before the sun goes down.** One of the best ways to clear Ama is to allow your body to detox naturally overnight. Your body is designed to cleanse and repair while you sleep. When you load it up with heavy evening meals, you expend all your precious resources on digestion. The more energy you use on digestion, the less you have for detoxing. I recommend eating a light evening meal, like soup or stew, before the sun goes down.

- **Satisfy your five senses.** Your body has five senses – sight, sound, hearing, touch and taste. Nourish these senses by only taking in what satisfies and delights you. You have the power to choose the energy you absorb. For example, you can choose to look at something, or not. You can choose to eat something, or not. If you hear something that doesn't serve you, let it go in one ear and out the other. You have more control over your environment than you might think!

- **Oil massage your body.** Oil is essential in Ayurveda. It provides vital lubrication to your body, bringing integrity through all seven layers of your skin. When you oil massage your body you soften your tissues, allowing toxic residues to be released. Oil massaging daily is best, but you could start by massaging once a week and build up from there. You can also protect yourself from harsh environmental factors, like office air conditioning, by dabbing some oil around your nostrils and in your ears.

- **Refresh your eyes and nose.** Splash some cold water on your eyes in the morning when you wake up. For the nose, consider trying a neti pot and salt rinses. You will love how clean and refreshed you feel!

- **Nurture your sense of taste.** There are two ways you can take care of your sense of taste. Tongue scraping is a wonderfully fast and effective option. You could also try oil pulling to keep your oral cavity clean.

~

I'm sure you'll agree that these practices are all incredibly fast, easy and affordable. Aside from investing in some oil, a neti pot and a tongue scraper, these practices don't cost a thing! There's no need to buy the latest Doshic teas and trending Ayurvedic treatments. All you need is a few key items that will not only help you heal, but also build a buffer of immunity. Isn't that a refreshing change? Especially if you're spending a fortune on clinical treatments. Of course, clinical treatments have their place. There may be times when you need clinical-grade herbs and professional treatments – but a monthly visit to your practitioner is wasted if you neglect daily practices at home. It's costly and disempowering to continually hand over the care of your body to someone else. Why not prevent the symptoms before they arise?

When it comes to managing your health, I believe it's the small daily details that make the biggest difference. By incorporating these simple Ama clearing practices into your day, you build your body's capacity to metabolise everything that enters your system through your five senses. This means your body is free to do what it does best – detox naturally! By clearing your body of toxic Ama, you create a healthy canvas to build on. This is when you can focus on Agni, which we'll get to in the next section. But first, let's address the elephant in the room.

At this point you might be wondering when we're going to talk about the popular Ayurvedic Doshas – Vata, Pitta and Kapha – and how Ama effects your body type. The reason why Ayurveda works is because it's tailored to you. It recognises your individuality, allowing you to develop a system that's as unique as you are. It's ironic then, that when most people discover Ayurveda, they immediately categorise themselves according to one of seven Dosha body types. Are you guilty of this?

The Doshas can be helpful to identify health conditions and categorise food groups, but they can also be extremely limiting. Every individual is beautifully unique and it's impossible to classify our diverse bodies by only three Doshas. If a questionnaire, or even a practitioner, identifies that you have a predominance in one of the Dosha categories, please note this most likely refers to your presenting state of health. It's not the essence of who you are. Your true body type is comprised of unchangeable aspects about your physicality, like how tall you are. Measuring it through questions about your moods or how often you poop in a day is not going to result in knowing your body type. You might have physical tendencies that fall into one category, but mental tendencies that fall into another. Stop trying to figure it out. Instead of getting caught up in the categorising system of the Doshas, realise that you've now entered the realm of Ayurveda, beyond the Doshas. Return to the bigger picture for more clarity – how the elements make up everything in the universe, including you.

THE ELEMENTS	TASTES	CONSTITUTION	SENSES
Ether	Bitter	Vata	Hearing
Air	Bitter, astringent, pungent	Vata	Touch
Fire	Pungent, sour, salty	Pitta	Sight
Water	Salty, sweet	Kapha Pitta	Taste
Earth	Sweet, sour, astringent	Kapha	Smell

Your body is built from the same five elements as other living things in nature – Space, Air, Fire, Water and Earth – albeit to varying degrees. Think about your bones. They're very light, they have holes in them. They have the element of space. Now think about the water in your body, the fire in your belly, the air in your lungs. The Earth element is present in everything that fills the gaps, including the muscle that holds up your very skeleton. Every element is there. From the subtle to the gross, your body tissue is sequentially developed and nourished. You are at one with the world around you. That's why, when you eat vegetables, your body recognises them as elemental nourishment it can digest, metabolize and assimilate to nourish your body tissues. It can't do this with processed food. You are so beautifully connected to nature!

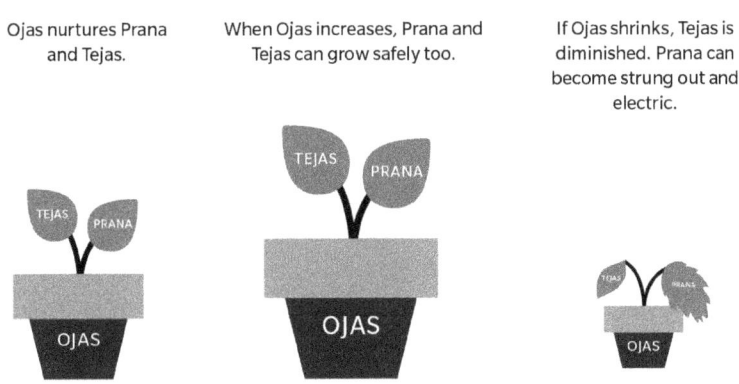

Ojas nurtures Prana and Tejas.

When Ojas increases, Prana and Tejas can grow safely too.

If Ojas shrinks, Tejas is diminished. Prana can become strung out and electric.

The governing forces of nature, the thing that makes your heart beat, we consider to be the life force called "Prana" in Ayurveda. This Prana works in conjunction with intelligence called "Tejas" and resources called "Ojas". You have all these energies inside you. We all do. It doesn't matter whether you are more Vata, Pitta or Kapha. Your body is brilliant by design. Ayurveda is about nurturing your natural brilliance by incorporating daily practices to help you look and feel your best. We'll navigate some more practical ways to do this in the next chapter, after some quick tips and exercises.

~

Self-care tip - Know your body beyond the Doshas.
To understand your body's constitution (called "Prakruti" in Ayurveda) beyond the limiting Dosha types, try the concept of "Panchmahabhuta" – the five elements. Thinking about your body in terms of the elements not only helps you to manage your health, it can also help you identify your duty –

your dharma – in life. The more you align your natural physicality to your work in this life, the healthier and happier you will be. For example, if you're physically earthy and solid, you may enjoy physical labour, like farming, gardening or cleaning. However, if you're naturally tall and thin, you may feel more at home in a design studio, an office or a shop. If you work in a role that's at odds with your body type, it's likely you'll become unwell. Find alignment wherever you can.

See how getting to know your body in terms of the elements provides more flexibility than the Doshas? Anyone can catch a cold or feel sad, not just Kapha types. Anyone can get sinusitis or feel angry, not just Pitta types. Similarly, anyone can suffer from dry skin or anxiety, not just Vata types. People love the Doshas because they are interesting and exotic, but they can perpetuate endless circling, with patients seeking remedies that simply won't work. This is what we're here to break free from! Instead of trying to determine your body "type" by changeable factors like mood or stool frequency, look to the elements. Think about your body holistically and consider all the inter-related factors that are contributing to your current condition. This holistic approach is the key to finding true balance.

Make a note: Think about your body and the type of work your physicality lends itself to. Does this align with your current role, or is there a conflict? Think about ways to create more connection and nurture your natural tendencies. If you're a strong, earthy type who feels stuck in an office all day, consider exercising at lunchtime or pitching the idea of a "walking meeting". Similarly, if you're light and airy, but your job is physically demanding, think about ways to rest and recharge. You could try taking a short nap in your break or wrapping yourself up in a cosy blanket for a quiet meditation. If you're really struggling with your work, brainstorm some new, exciting options. What type of work would you love to do that would make you feel happy and well?

Self-care tip - Align with the Cycle of Life.
Ayurveda is based on the theory that everything is born, exists and dies. We call these three phases of activity the three "Gunas". The first Guna is "Sattva", which refers to a state of creation. It's about being light and blissful. "Rajas" is a state of motion, where the mind is vibrant and active. "Tamas" means to perish. When things don't cycle this natural way, it means there's trouble in the body. There'll be Ama that needs to be cleared. Waste

products called "Malas" need to be removed from your system at a cellular level. This happens in many ways – from breathing to crying tears, sneezing, burping and passing wind. When natural urges arise in your body, remember they're "better out than in".

You can ensure the life force in you cycles in flow by simply tuning in to your body. As well as honouring your natural urges, ask your body how it feels and give yourself what you need. Think about adjectives that describe how you're feeling and counter them with opposites (these adjectives are called "gunas", which we'll be exploring shortly). For example, if you feel cold, it's probably not wise to drink a cold milkshake. A warming one-pot wonder might be a better option. Similarly, if you feel sad, sombre music probably won't help. Uplifting sounds and sunshine are more likely to do the trick. In Ayurveda, like attracts like. When you want to clear toxic Ama, do the opposite of how you feel. Let's try it right now.

Make a note: Take a moment to check in with your body. What emotions do you feel? Are you hot, cold, tired, anxious? Now, think of some ways you could feel better. Write them all down, then choose one to do in the next hour. If you're feeling tired and flat, you may not feel like going for a walk, but try it and see how you go. Notice if you feel more balanced by the time you get back. No matter how busy you feel, make body checks a priority. Even walking for just a minute or two will feel deeply supportive to your body and mind. You'll be amazed at how you can turn things around and create incredible space to heal.

THE DAILY WAY
If you're not regenerating, you're degenerating.
Rejuvenate with Dinacharya.

I mentioned that learning how your body works would be a two-step process. We've already covered the first step – how to clear Ama. Now let's move on to the next step – how to increase Agni. Agni refers to digestive capacity. It's kryptonite to Ama. When you loosen Ama and eliminate it with Agni, what's left is clarity – the key to lasting health and happiness. That's what Bold Freedom is all about.

In this section, you'll learn how to increase your body's Agni so you can shine from the inside out. We'll be expanding on the daily practices, Dinacharya, adding exciting new tools and rituals into your arsenal. But before we begin, I'd like to introduce you to what we call the "Koshas" in Ayurveda. Understanding the Koshas will help you better understand how and why Dinacharya works and provide context throughout this section. As with everything in Bold Freedom, I want to empower you with enough theory to satisfy your thirst for knowledge, without drowning you in the details! I'm sure you'll find the Koshas fascinating.

~

There are five Koshas in Ayurveda, which represent aspects of your complete self. They are:

- **Annamaya Kosha** – your food body
- **Pranamaya Kosha** – your breath body
- **Manomaya Kosha** – your mental body
- **Vijnanamaya Kosha** – your intuitive body
- **Anandamaya Kosha** – your bliss body

Think of the Koshas as sheaths or energetic layers. Like Chakras, Koshas have their own individual functions, but they aren't the same as Chakras. Imagine the Chakras like energy centres aligned vertically along your spine. Spiralling out from these Chakras are "Nadi" channels where your life force pulsates. You may have also heard of "Srotas" – the thirteen channels, like pores on your skin, where your body takes in energy and expels waste. It's important to keep these channels clean to prevent Ama build up. Ayurveda is a vast science, with many complex terms and specialised streams. While it's helpful and interesting to study these, we want to keep things simple. The aim is to align your body and mind in your environment, because it's here that you'll relax into easeful living, allowing health and happiness to bloom. Understanding the Koshas is critical to achieving this, so let's delve into them.

The Koshas layer from the deepest, most internal parts of your spiritual body to the most external aspects of your physical body. Imagine them starting down in your spine, deep within your nervous system, and running all the way through to the outermost layer of your skin. From here, they extend even further, from your physical form outward, as you expand into breath and eventually become blissfully one with the world around you.

Your Koshas embody every aspect of YOU – your beautiful, complex, five-layered being – and all five need to be nourished. With a little care and thought, it's possible to feed every sheath simultaneously, by considering both the internal and external factors that impact wellbeing. Let's use the act of eating, for example. When we think about eating, the Annamaya Kosha, the food body, immediately springs to mind, However, when you eat with health in mind, you can make all your Koshas sing.

- **Your food body** can be satisfied by eating clean, nourishing, natural food at optimum times of the day.
- **Your breath body** can be satisfied by breathing three times deeply before each meal (a bonus Ayurveda tip!)
- **Your mental body** can be satisfied by planning and scheduling your meals, so you feel organised and relaxed.
- **Your intuitive body** can be satisfied by eating fruits and vegetables that are in-season.
- **Your bliss body** can be satisfied by choosing foods you love and sharing a meal with your family.

See how everything works together? Keep this in mind as we explore some more specific ways to improve Agni through Dinacharya. The practical application will look different for everyone. However, if you find a way to feed all your five Koshas at once, you know you're onto a winning thing!

~

STEP 9 IMPROVE AGNI
In Ayurveda we follow a daily routine based on how our bodies are designed to function and thrive. This is how we improve Agni, allowing us to digest all incoming substances – and avoid accumulating Ama. The principles of this daily routine, called Dinacharya, are guidelines for healthy living. They help us align to circadian rhythms and the natural cycles in our body, so we can rejuvenate as we get older. They literally help us to age gracefully!

The Dinacharya guidelines are based on the Grandmother wisdom and respect for precious resources like time, energy and food. No one teaches us this anymore. Mainstream wellbeing today is all about "quick fixes" and "miracle cures". But you know from experience these don't work. That's why you're here, reading Bold Freedom. As you create your own daily routine and dedicate time to feel well, you'll develop your own wisdom. This wisdom is your life-long ticket to health and happiness. Once you learn it, it's yours for life. It's the greatest gift you can give to yourself!

The Dinacharya guidelines can be very detailed and there are different interpretations. To make things as easy as possible, I'll start by outlining the key elements, together with some practical scenarios. I'll then give an example of the Dinacharya in action, showing how they might look in your day.

~

Food
How and when you nourish your body is a fundamental element of Dinacharya. We've talked about diet in previous chapters, so let's quickly recap what we've already covered:
- Limit eating outside daylight hours
- Eat your largest meal at lunchtime
- Eat an early, light dinner before the sun goes down

- Choose whole, seasonal, plant-based foods
- Prepare your food as freshly as possible (avoid pre-cooking and freezing)
- Incorporate the six tastes (sweet, sour, salty, bitter, astringent and pungent) in every meal

If you can master these basics, you'll be well on your way to a clearer head, a healthier gut, a happier mind and a lighter body. However, when you're ready to boost your routine, there are many more things you can do to fire up your digestion.

The first is to eat with the seasons. Choosing in-season foods is a key way to work with your body's intelligence and harness the powerful forces of nature (and nourish your intuitive body!). Think about where your food comes from and how it grows. Leafy green plants like spinach and kale reach up and out, capturing the sun. When you eat those plants, it's almost like you're eating sunshine. Your body is flooded with vitamins, antioxidants and chlorophyll, which helps cleanse your blood and detox your body. These are perfect in the warmer weather. Then you have root vegetables that sit in the ground, like carrots and potatoes. There's a reason why these sweet, heavy vegetables are so nourishing in winter. They are exactly what your body needs and what it is designed to have!

A second tip is to spice up your meals. In Ayurveda, herbs and spices are like superfoods. They contain an array of antioxidants and nutrients – both the fresh and dried varieties. Try incorporating more herbs and spices into your meals, particularly the bitter, pungent and astringent tastes we often lack in Western food. As you begin to appreciate herbs and spices – even the basics like salt and pepper – you'll discover what your body loves. You'll intuitively know what your body craves, and so will the people you cook for. Imagine asking your family, "Do you feel like oregano on the pasta or would you like black pepper?" Some family members will say "both", some will say "just oregano" or "just pepper". How wonderful to see your whole family tap into their health and delight in their meals. This is a gift you can give!

Another way to level up your food game is to simply eat a little less. Not just for dinner, but overall. If you're fit for it, you can dive right in here and reduce your dinner tonight but if not, go easy over time developing a cleaner, lighter way of fuelling your body. You want to avoid waking hungry in the night. Food is often used to compensate, soothe or reward. I noticed this particularly when travelling in Europe and Asia, where the entire day is centred around food. If you examine your eating habits, you'll probably find you eat emotionally. Yet physically you need very little to thrive. In fact, when your nervous systems are lulled, your Agni functions at its best. You absorb the bioavailable nutrition from food more readily. However, when you fire up your bodies with large, heavy meals, you also fire up your nervous systems. It's like putting a water extinguisher on your digestive fire!

Make a note: Have you ever kept a food diary? Writing out what, when and how you eat can be daunting but enlightening. Try keeping a food diary for a few days, recording everything you eat. Make a note about how you feel before and after each meal. How is your energy? Do you feel satisfied? Is your hunger emotional or physical? Are you eating in-season foods? Are you eating too much? As you start implementing healthier habits, you can compare how different foods make you feel. Once patients start a food diary, I often ask them to go back and try a food they have been avoiding. This can lead to some surprises! For example, a cold, sweet smoothie for breakfast can often cause a "3pm slump", but patients don't recognise this until they keep track. They believe they are making a healthy choice, until they do a body check and think about how that smoothie makes them feel. In most cases, it only takes a few days to notice the effects.

A final tip for nailing your nutrition is to eat intuitively and easefully. When you're mapping out your meals for the week, keep it simple and don't be tempted to follow trends thinking every "health food" you see must be good for you. Remember, everybody has different needs. We respond uniquely to certain foods. For example, not everyone has bile that can deal with naturally occurring salicylates. Some people break out in a rash if they eat strawberries. The berry-loaded acai bowls, which are so popular on social media, would be a very bad choice for these people! The best thing to do is to listen to your body and go back to those descriptive adjectives. Nourish yourself with foods you enjoy and make meals that fit your budget and lifestyle – this includes what works for your family. The easier and more enjoyable your meal plan, the more likely it is that you'll stick to it!

~

Movement
Our bodies are designed to move. To move is to be alive. Movement is essential for our blood to circulate, oxygen to reach our cells and nutrients

to be absorbed. It also allows the heavy mass we don't need to pass out (through sweat, bowel movements, tears etc) so we can feel light and vibrant. Without movement we get stuck. Think about an old car. If you leave a car sitting in front of your house without turning the engine over, it will not start. Your body is the same.

There will be times when movement feels difficult or impossible, but please keep moving any way you can. Even the smallest breath sweeping through the body reflects a wave of movement. It means that you are still alive and sometimes gentle movement is the best. I remember waking up one morning. I wanted to get up, but I couldn't move my body. I felt so weak but I knew I had to keep moving, to get up for the children. I lay for a while, focusing everything I had on my body, taking slow, smooth breaths. As life returned, my mind and body reconnected with a new understanding of my limits. I decided not to let myself wear out again. The same can happen for you if you're stuck. Keep moving every day. You can start small with simple breathing exercises, then build up to yoga or walking. The more you move, the easier it will become.

~

Sleep
We talked previously about the power of sleep to detox your body. Sleep is essential for reducing Ama and also increasing Agni. If you want to bounce out of bed in the morning, follow the sleep routine below, which we covered in chapter one.

- Start winding down by 8.30pm. Dim the lights and kill the screens.
- Nourish yourself with an oil massage about half an hour before bed, focusing on your feet and give yourself a weekly head massage for the best night's sleep!
- Take some time for quiet reflection, leaving any negative thoughts behind.
- Be asleep by the latest 10pm.
- Rise at the same time every morning, even on the weekends.

Try this for three days and see how your body feels. If this is very different to your current routine, it may take a few days to adjust. The good news is, you've already taken steps to make the transition easier. By mapping your time out in your calendar and planning your meals, you've got a head start on tomorrow. Plus, by eating a lighter evening meal, you're setting your body up for success. You might even experience a sensation you haven't felt since you were a child – waking up feeling hungry. When you wake up feeling hungry, it means your metabolism has aligned. Your body has processed your nutrition overnight and is ready to rid the waste. That's how you want to feel in the morning. Light, free and refreshed. It beats waking up tired, puffy and groggy – then chasing your tail all day! You'll feel more rested when you sleep according to your body clock more than if you sleep in for hours.

Of course, there are times when your body needs more sleep, like when you've had a busy week or you're recovering from illness. Follow your sleep routine as often as you can but listen to your body when it speaks. Some days you may need a slower paced morning or an extra hour sleep, so go to bed earlier. The key is to feel restful when you're sleeping, not guilty. You know what your body needs.

~

Oil and Water
We touched on oil in the previous section. Oil is a fundamental element of Dinacharya. It cleans your body and nourishes your tissues with life-giving health. Imagine an oil molecule surrounding a toxin that's inside your body. Oil absorbs and isolates all the goodness, sucking nourishment deep into your skin. Everything toxic is left behind, so it can be expelled and rinsed off. By bringing connectivity to all the seven layers of your skin, oil clears the conversation between the cells in your body, so its natural intelligence can function more highly. The benefits are mind-blowing!
Oil also provides essential hydration. Think about oil like water. Have you ever noticed the more water you drink throughout the day, the thirstier you feel? You may not notice how dry your body feels, but that doesn't mean you don't need to oil. The more you oil your body, the more nourishing benefits you'll feel. You won't know until you try it, then you'll see what you've been missing!
The same applies to water. Dryness is the body's enemy. Dehydration and constipation deplete the body, leading to auto-immune conditions, congestion and chronic diseases. These diseases impact one in three people. You don't want to be one of them! Hydrate your body by sipping water, particularly warm water, throughout the day.

Meditation

Meditation helps quieten your mind, allowing you to think more clearly. It's an important part of Dinacharya. When your mind is sharp and clear, you can respond to situations with poise, rather than reacting out of fear. We talked about this in chapter one.

If you're looking for a way to nourish all five Koshas simultaneously, look no further than meditation. Let me explain how meditation connects you to every part of being and gives life to your Koshas.

- By taking a few minutes to become aware of your breath when you wake in the morning, you give life to your Pranamaya Kosha – your breath body.
- By pausing and steadying yourself before you walk out the door in the morning, you nourish your Manomaya Kosha – your mental body.
- When you reflect quietly on your day and notice what made you feel good, you connect with your Vijnanamaya Kosha – the intuitive body.
- You can even nourish your Annamaya Kosha – food body – by breathing deeply three times before you eat, as I described earlier.
- As you use meditation to create a connection between all these aspects of yourself, you tap into your Anandamaya Kosha – your bliss body.

Remember I said if you can find a way to feed all five Koshas at once, you know you're onto a good thing? Meditation is a very good thing! Whether you're a seasoned meditator or you're just starting out, this practice has the power to change your life. Plus, you can do it any way you like, anywhere you like. You might choose to attend a meditation class or download one of the many guided meditation apps. Or you could just sit quietly in your home, your car, or even out in public once you learn to quieten your mind. Meditation truly is the world's most versatile practice!

Dinacharya in Action

Now you understand the core elements of Dinacharya, I want to show you how easy it is to incorporate them into your day. Below is an example of a daily routine, with morning, afternoon and evening practices.

Morning routine

1. **Pause.** When you first wake up, take a moment to lie in bed. Become aware of your physical body. Now, take a few deep breaths and tune into your spiritual body. Notice the energy force of prana cycling within you. All you need to do is notice.

2. **Hydrate.** Once you're up and you've passed urine, drink one to two glasses of warm water. This will help you pass a stool and eliminate some of the Ama your body naturally starts to re-absorb about three minutes after you wake up.

3. **Eliminate.** Hopefully you'll be ready to pass a stool. If you're not, don't worry. The time will come later in the morning. You may also need to pass a second stool around 2:30pm when the natural energies bring verve to your body. If you're at work or school, you may not feel comfortable passing a stool. Your body wants to feel relaxed and open, so it may contract until you get home. Again, that's OK. The main thing is that you eliminate every 24 hours.

4. **Refresh.** It's now time to splash a bit of cold water on your eyes, scrape your tongue and brush your teeth. If you want to oil pull, go ahead.

5. **Oil.** I now recommend oiling your body. Have a special space where you can perform this ritual and oil your body from head to toe.

6. **Move.** I know you've just oiled your body but consider putting on some old exercise clothes and creating a little sweat. Some people prefer to move first, then oil, then shower. However, if you oil first, the sweat from movement will help the oil remove toxins from your body. Once you've had a shower, apply some more oil as a moisturiser.

7. **Breathe.** If you have time for a morning meditation, do that before you leave home. Even if you're pressed for time, you can do a simple breathing exercise where you use your thumb and index finger to block one nostril at a time. Alternate breathing between your right and your left nostril, keeping the other one closed. Even ten or twenty breaths can help steady you for the day. You will be surprised at how effective this is!

8. **Eat.** Have a nourishing, healthy breakfast made from natural whole-

foods. Don't make it a large meal – just enough to get you through to lunch without needing to snack. If you're preparing your lunch before you leave home, do that now too.

Midday routine

1. **Eat.** Enjoy your freshly made lunch, around midday if you can. Make this your largest meal of the day, so you don't need to snack before dinner.

2. **Move.** If you can, do some light movement after lunch to help your body with digestion. A brisk walk around the block is the perfect way to spend your lunch break. Better than scrolling on your phone!

Evening routine

1. **Eat.** Consume a light, early dinner. Keep it simple, fresh and delicious. Incorporate as many herbs and spices as you like and try to include all six tastes.

2. **Enjoy.** Now's the time to do something joyful. Reward yourself for your efforts today with anything you love to do. Read a book, watch a movie, do some knitting, or walk your dog. Finding this time is so much easier when you have an early dinner.

3. **Relax.** Begin preparing your body for sleep by winding down around 8.30pm. Dim the lights, turn off your screens and start preparing for bed.

4. **Oil.** Oil your entire body again, paying special attention to your feet. Rub oil over every part of your feet, from your heels to your toes.

5. **Meditate.** Take a few precious moments to reflect on the day and sit quietly with yourself. You could listen to a guided meditation or simply sit in stillness. Do whatever works for you.

6. **Sleep.** Be asleep by 10pm so you can wake feeling wonderful tomorrow.

~

I hope you can see how easy it is to make Ayurveda part of your day. The above example of Dinacharya is a guide to show you how your day might look. However, you don't have to be rigid. When you're rigid, everything scrapes up against you. That's not the way to feel better. You want to be more like a tree. Have your roots firmly planted in the ground but have a degree of flexibility. Remember, Bold Freedom is about discovering what makes you feel better and simply doing more of that. It's about establishing positive habits that become non-negotiables in your day – creating the consistency that's been lacking in your previous wellbeing efforts.

Pick and choose the practices that work for you. And, if you feel overwhelmed, just start with one or two. Keep it simple. Take my morning routine, for example. Every morning I move my body, mind and soul before breakfast. It's that easy. I tune into my body, listen to what it needs, then do that. It could be yoga, a walk, or sitting outside in the sun. It usually takes between thirty and sixty minutes and it's completely spontaneous. If you're the kind of person who likes to feel free and impulsive, why not try this for yourself? What could be more spontaneous than giving your body what it needs in that exact moment? That's the ultimate freedom!

~

Want to go a little deeper? The beauty of Ayurveda is that there are so many layers to explore. Dinacharya is the daily way to detox and cleanse your system, but there are ways to experience a deeper cleanse in line with the seasons. In Ayurveda, we use the term "Ritucharya" to describe seasonal adjustments to our daily routine. Ritucharya allows your "Mahavahasrota", the main channel of your gut, to get a complete reset. It involves lifestyle and diet modification to help your body copy with the physical and mental impacts of the seasons.

Even though there are four seasons, you don't need to experience Ritucharya four times a year. Twice a year is optimum, with spring and autumn being the best times. In spring, the aim of Ritucharya is to rid your body of the heaviness, weight and mucus from winter. In autumn, you want to focus on expelling some of the summer heat.

A good way to approach Ritucharya is to avoid adjectives that describe the season you're leaving behind. Instead, focus on adjectives that describe the season you're heading into. For example, if you're leaving behind a cold, wet season you want to avoid cold, wet things. If you're heading into a warm, dry season, favour warm, light foods. See yourself as part of nature and do what the plants are doing.

Another method you can use, if you're interested in exploring Ritucharya, is to look at the Ayurvedic gunas. The gunas I am referring to here are not the three Gunas we discussed in the previous section (Sattvas, Rajas and Tamas). These gunas are twenty qualities (10 pairs of opposites) that help you understand your body. These are the adjectives we touched on earlier to describe how your body is feeling. They are the cornerstones of Ayurveda – the fundamentals from which treatment plans and remedies are devised – and they can be used for any daily or seasonal routines. They are:

ATTRIBUTE/GUNA

Heavy/guru	Oily/snigdha	Soft/mrudu	Clear/vishada
Light/laghu	Dry/ruksha	Hard/kathina	Cloudy/avila
Slow, dull/manda	Slimy/shlakshna	Static, stable/sthira	Sticky/picchila
Sharp/tikshna	Rough/khara	Mobile/chala	
Cold/shita	Dense, concentrated/sandra	Subtle/sukshma	
Hot/ushna	Liquid, dilute/drava	Gross/sthula	

- Heavy – Light
- Slow – Sharp
- Cold – Hot
- Oily – Dry
- Smooth – Rough
- Dense – Liquid
- Static – Mobile
- Gross – Subtle
- Cloudy – Clear

These sensations, or gunas, can be applied to anything you experience. Think about how happiness feels – light, mobile and clear. Sadness, on the other hand, feels heavy, static and cloudy. When you think of your physical body in terms of the gunas, you can find a natural remedy for almost any ailment. For example, if your body is feeling dry (think flaky skin and rashes), try oiling and drinking more water. If you're experiencing wetness and heaviness in the form of a cough, try drinking some warm, sharp ginger tea. Or sit outside in the dry sun. See how your body tells you the answers? Now you're starting to take notice! Using the gunas is so much easier than trying to fathom the Doshic needs of your body. Bold Freedom is all about ease and the gunas are an invaluable tool!

~

Tip you can try today - Choose health.
As you develop your daily routine, think of every element as a choice. Instead of saying "I can't eat chocolate" or "I'm not allowed to eat chocolate", try saying "I CHOOSE not to eat chocolate". Because you CAN eat chocolate, if you choose. Bold Freedom is about doing more things that make you feel better and crowding out things that don't. It's about consistency, not perfection. If you choose to eat nourishing food all week, you can choose to eat chocolate now and then. This choice can be guilt free. How wonderfully refreshing!

Tip you can try today - Combat food cravings.
When it comes to food cravings, there are two types – those that come from your "well self" that knows what your body REALLY wants, and those that come from your "unwell self" that wants to feed existing imbalances. If you regularly crave unhealthy foods, this is likely your "unwell self" talking. The more you listen to your voice of wellness, the quieter your unhealthy voice will become. The next time you feel a craving, ask yourself which type it is. If it's a healthy craving, satisfy it. If it's unhealthy, recognise it – then make a choice, as mentioned above. As you learn more about your body and understand the "why behind the why", you'll find it easier to make healthy choices.

Tip you can try today - Respect your age.
Age is no barrier to health, but it should be respected. As you venture through Bold Freedom, remember to do what feels right for you TODAY. Jogging may have felt good years ago, but it might not today. If it doesn't feel good, don't do it – no matter how "trendy" something is, or how much you think you "should" be doing it! Don't push yourself or ignore your body when it gives you feedback. Your body changes all the time. Love and accept it every day.

Tip you can try today - Alleviate Menstural or Hormonal issues.

If you suffer from female reproductive issues, there are two practices than can ease your symptoms – and we've covered them both in this chapter. The first one is oiling your body. Oil combats dryness that comes from a surge in reproductive hormones. Say goodbye to dry skin forever! The second is the breathing method I described earlier, where you breathe through one nostril at a time. This calms the nervous system, releases tension and reduces the stress hormone, cortisol.

FOUR: ENJOY THE PRACTICE

CHANGING DIRECTION AND TROUBLESHOOTING

You've set goals, made time and space, and created an actionable plan for success. You've even begun to clear blocks and implement daily wellbeing practices. On paper, things look perfect – but we all know that "life happens". Sometimes even the best laid plans don't pan out the way we'd like. Challenges arise, things pop up, life takes unexpected twists. That's all part of the fun!

As you journey through Bold Freedom, you're bound to encounter some obstacles. While you can't control life's events, you can control how you respond to them – and I want to show you how. In this chapter, I'll share some tips to help make the transition to your new lifestyle as smooth and stress-free as possible. I'll also talk through some troubleshooting strategies you can use when life gets in the way. So, instead of giving up, you can keep moving forward – all while staying true to your goals, your values, and your vision. Let's start with some simple tips.

~

Top tips for your Bold Freedom journey.
Just start
No matter where you're starting from, or how far away your goals seem, the important thing is to just begin. You've already set a date in your calendar, so be true and stick to it. The first days and weeks are the most important when it comes to forming new habits, so commit to the promises you've made. Change can't begin until you do.

Keep showing up

Remember my recipe for success? Intuition and consistency. If you follow the plan you've intuitively created and commit to showing up every day, your success is almost a certainty. Change happens gradually, so you may not notice the subtle shifts. However, if you show up daily throughout the quarter, I guarantee you'll see results. Be patient and trust the process.

Don't edit while you write

No one can predict the future, so why waste precious energy trying? Think about your journey like writing a book. You can't edit a book you haven't written yet. If you try to edit as you write, you end up going around in circles and never getting past the first chapter. Get through the first draft (the first quarter), without getting weighed down by details. Once the first draft is done, you can reflect on your progress. You can tweak, refine and reset with a much clearer mind.

If you constantly feel the urge to edit your plan, it could be a sign that fear is creeping in. The good news is, you'll see it coming. You've done the work. You know the signs. You have the tools to overcome. Just stay strong, stick to your plan, and remember why you started this journey. You're tired of going in circles, right?

Get comfortable being uncomfortable

There's no getting around the fact that change can be uncomfortable. The bigger the change, the more uncomfortable things can be. But this is a sign of growth. It means you're outside your comfort zone, which is where life really begins!

If you start feeling overwhelmed, put things into perspective. No matter how uncomfortable things get, I bet you've lived through much worse. Plus, if you REALLY want to quit, the option is there. Take solace in that. You can choose to quit anytime, but is that what you really want? Do you really want to give up on your dreams or is that just fear talking? You'll know the answer when the question arises.

Check-in constantly with your calendar

Your quarterly calendar is your roadmap to success. Refer to it regularly. No matter how clear you feel about the path you've carved out, you can't have too much reinforcement. Look at your calendar every day to get a big picture view of your day, your week, your month and your quarter. Wrap your head around your weekly actions each Sunday, so you feel poised and prepared on Monday morning. Have you ever heard the saying, "You get what you focus on, so focus on what you want"? You have everything you want mapped out. Focus on it and bring it to life!

Always follow your intuition
Information is understanding, whereas knowledge arises from within. Wisdom is garnered from the experience of where information and understanding meet. In Bold Freedom, I'm giving you lots of information. However, you already have the innate knowledge of what your body wants and needs. You hold the key to your health and happiness. Tap into your Vijnanamaya Kosha and do what feels RIGHT. I recommend checking in with yourself every 24 hours, ideally in the evening before bed, and asking yourself "what worked today?" Learn what makes your body feel good and commit to doing more of that.

Trust yourself to experiment
The more you use your intuition, the more you'll learn to trust yourself. This will give you the freedom and confidence to experiment. Try something new to eat. Move your body in a new way. Do something totally different. Every time you try something new, reflect on how it made you feel and choose if you want to do it again. Over time, you'll develop your own personal toolkit of things that make you feel great, like going for a walk when you feel overwhelmed, or starting your day with some sun salutations. Play the wonderful game of life! You won't know what works until you try.

Be kind to yourself
Remember we talked about being your own best friend? Your inner dialogue and the words you use influence how you feel and behave. Please be kind to yourself! Talk to yourself encouragingly and notice the nuances in your language. You'll be surprised at how the tiniest shift can totally change a sentence's meaning. For example, instead of saying "I'm anxious" or "I'm hopeless", try saying "I FEEL anxious" or "I FEEL hopeless". It's more than OK to feel emotions, but don't define yourself by them. Negative feelings will come and go. Focus more on your actions, as these are what lead to results.

Be kind to others
As you tread the Bold Freedom waters, be mindful of how your actions im-

pact others. Communicate openly, share honestly, and connect consciously with the people around you. You'll soon discover that positivity attracts positivity. Be a magnet for good vibes, even on a bad day.

Live without regrets

Life is full of opportunities. If you have a bad day, or you venture off track, please don't berate yourself. We all have times where we wish we'd said or did something differently. It can be tempting to replay these moments in your head, thinking "Why did I do that?" or "If only I'd said this". No matter how significant something seems, it rarely matters in the big scheme of things. Yes, you want to "live in the moment", but you don't want to live in it twice! What happened in the past doesn't matter. What matters is now. What are you going to do NOW? Let's talk troubleshooting tactics.

~

Troubleshooting Strategies

Learning how to deal with difficult days is an essential part of Bold Freedom. Say you miss your morning exercise session, or a family emergency pops up on spring cleaning day. How can you practically navigate life's curveballs without completely derailing your plans? Below are some of my favourite strategies for obliterating overwhelm, managing time, and staying on track when times get tough. I hope you find these helpful.

Don't make time that doesn't exist

So, you've missed something important on your schedule. It's not ideal, but it is OK. My number one tip in this situation is to simply do whatever's next. Just move on with your day, instead of trying to play catch up. When you try to squeeze in extra tasks, you risk pushing others out. This creates a domino effect that can throw your whole day off track. Before you know it, you'll be back to where you started, before you even had a calendar!

If you have lots of white space in your day, you may choose to catch up. The main thing is to be practical. The worst-case scenario is that you'll need to reschedule, but that might motivate you even more. You'll be raring to do that task you've missed at the next available time. At the very least, you'll learn something about how you feel when things don't go to plan. Whether that's noticing how rigid your body feels without exercise, or how much you prefer to work at a clean desk, every learning is a win.

Learn to prioritise
Things go wrong all the time, but not everything requires immediate action. When something unexpected pops up, try categorising it in terms of urgency and importance. There's a tool called the "Eisenhower Matrix" that can help you do this easily by rating tasks from one to four. This is how it looks:

Level 1: Urgent and important – DO
Level 2: Important, but not urgent – PLAN
Level 3: Urgent, but not important – DELEGATE
Level 4: Not urgent and not important – ELIMINATE

The Eisenhower Matrix is used often in business, but it works just as well for Bold Freedom. If something is urgent and important, it's OK to tend to it now. If it's important, but not urgent, find time for it in your weekly plan but don't derail your plans for the day. If something is urgent but not important, think about who you could delegate to. Finally, if something is not urgent and not important, simply eliminate it. It's OK to let things go. You have permission to be imperfect, especially when it comes to menial tasks. Save your energy for things that matter.

The brilliant thing about your calendar is that you've built white space into it. You also have a three-hour strategic block each week, where you can reshuffle and add new tasks. You are supported by the system you've created, so lean comfortably into that! Sit on things for a day or two, rather than reacting out of fear. I recommend having a holding place for things or ideas, so you don't lose track. You could use the notes section of your digital calendar, a written "to-do" list, a whiteboard, or sticky notes. Whatever helps you stay on track. It's all about organisation!

Accept the things you cannot change
Have you ever had one of those days where nothing seems to go to plan? When your mind is spinning, your heart is racing, and the whole world seems to conspire against you? Maybe you get stuck in traffic, assigned an urgent project, or the kids come down with a sudden sickness. Maybe all three things happen at once! The best thing to do in these situations is to slow down and get outside your own head. Become "the observer" of your situation, like an outsider looking in. From the position of observer, you can accept the things you cannot change. What could you possibly do about traffic? How could you control what happens at work? Some days you need

to be flexible. Be light-hearted if you can, because today's problems rarely matter tomorrow.

- **Consult your secret "Board of Directors"**

You have the power to change your plans. With daily check-ins, weekly plans and big quarterly resets, Bold Freedom gives you plenty of chances to readjust. That said, you can't expect to constantly change and have the method hold up. So how do you decide when it's right to change or when you should stay the course? One strategy you can try is to create a secret Board of Directors.

Think of three people you admire – the people you'd call if you were on a quiz show and needed help with a question. They could be famous people, historical figures, or people from your own life. When you're grappling with a decision, ask the Board. What would they would do in your position? If you could sit with them at the table, which way would they vote? By removing yourself just one degree from a decision, you give yourself space to think more objectively. Again, you become the observer.

- **Don't be afraid to ask for help**

You have so many resources, talents and skills. One of those skills is to ask for help. If you're really struggling with a decision, or you need support in a specific area, don't be afraid to seek support. The imaginary Board of Directors is great, but real people are even better. Talk to your family, friends and colleagues, and troubleshoot problems together.

When you reach out for help there are no guarantees. However, most people are happy to help when they can. And, really, what have you got to lose? Even if someone doesn't have the time or resources, at least you'll be on their radar. Say it's your boss, for example. They may not be able to help with THIS project, but they might think twice before allocating the next one.

- **Make time for self-care**

When life gets super busy, self-care is one of the first things to slip. Ironically, these are the times when you need it the most. Think about your health like a bank. If you keep making withdrawals and never deposit, you're left with an empty balance. You end up depleted, exhausted and prone to illness. I know this from personal experience. Here's a case study from my own life, which highlights the importance of self-care.

Case Study: Me!
Just recently, I struggled through one of the most demanding weeks of my life. Work was incredibly busy, I had lots happening at home, plus I was writing this book. I increased my output to meet the demands, but I didn't prioritise self-care. I made too many withdrawals from my bank of health and not nearly enough deposits. I clearly recall one day where I didn't make time to hydrate. It was 2pm before I realised I'd barely sipped any water all day. Knowing that dehydration and stress can attract colds, I went into damage control. I drank more water and oil massaged my body. However, I didn't sleep or rest the way that was needed. I kept going for a few more days, overdrawing my bank further. By day four, I was craving lollies, which made me feel even more lethargic. I drank extra water and went for bike ride, but even that didn't invigorate me. It was only when I found myself lying on the floor, completely exhausted, that I realised a cold was on its way.

At this point, I had two choices. I could CHOOSE to get a cold or I could CHOOSE self-care. The decision was a no-brainer. I looked at my calendar to see how I could reshuffle my week, prioritising the pressing items. I drank more water, oiled my body more often, and ventured outside on my bike daily. I also said "no" to late nights, so I could prioritise sleep by 10pm. It wasn't necessarily easy or convenient to make these changes, but I chose to hold this space for myself. And guess what? Within two days, I felt better. I caught that cold before it caught me!

~

I hope these tips bring you comfort and confidence. No matter what challenges you encounter on your journey, you have the power to surpass them. It all comes down to planning and organisation – making the time to live well. While this may seem rigorous on the surface, it's part of the recipe for success. Think of your Bold Freedom plan as a solid platform which you can launch from. You can wander, thrive and experience all of life's possibilities, knowing you have a stable base. You can be creative and spontaneous, yet also secure, knowing your body is well cared for and your health is in-check. What could be more freeing than that?

Self-care tip you can try today - Deep belly breathing.
While you can't control what happens in life, you can almost always control your breath. Deep belly breathing is a self-care strategy that's available to

you anytime, anywhere – and the benefits are phenomenal. This beautiful practice settles your nervous system, stimulates the relaxation response, and physiologically changes your body. You can try it right now. Sit, stand or lie down, keeping your spine straight. Now take slow, deep breaths into your belly – inhale for four counts, exhale for four counts. Feel your belly rise and fall. Notice your rib cage expand and contract. Keep going with this practice and experience a wave of calm wash over you. It can take as little as three breaths. That's a total of 24 seconds!

SHARE WHAT YOU HAVE, RINSE AND REPEAT
You are graced with strength and vitality.
Share your gifts, then receive some more.

As your physical health increases, you'll notice your mental capacity broaden and deepen. Get ready for an amazing ride! The capacity of your mind is beyond comprehension and you may have only scratched the surface. Have you ever noticed that when you wear a blue shirt, everyone around you seems to be wearing blue? Maybe they wear blue every day, but you don't notice until you tune in. This is because your mind and your senses are designed to take in only what you can fathom. Now that you understand how your body works, imagine how much more you can receive?

You're tuned into the right frequency now, so focus on what you'd like to see in your world. Put health and happiness on your radar and watch how the universe works for you. Energy flows where your attention goes. People, places and things will pop up like magic, manifesting in many ways. You might find a farmer's market in your local area, or stumble across a new yoga studio. Perhaps you'll meet a new friend or teacher to support you on your wellness journey. When your eyes are open to new possibilities, you see new rays of sunshine and light. And you know what's even better? You too can be a beacon of light for people around you.

By becoming more self-aware, you can share your gifts, spread good vibes, and gently guide others to greatness. However, the trick is to tread carefully. As you begin to feel the benefits of Bold Freedom, you might be tempted to tell everybody. It's natural to want your loved ones to feel healthier and happier – especially if you see them struggling and you feel you've found a solution. Just be mindful that not everyone is ready for change. Think about how long it took you to embrace change. Did you reach that tipping point, where the fear of staying the same became too much to bear? How long did you struggle on your own beaten path before you could even consider another possibility? Remember, everyone is on their own journey. So, while you may have people's best interests at heart, you don't want to push anyone out of their comfort zone. Respect their boundaries, honour their uniqueness, and have compassion for their fragility.

The best thing you can do is lead by example. When your loved ones see you thriving, they'll probably want to know what your secret is! They may ask you for advice or show interest in this book you're reading – but let them create change in their own time. It needs to be their decision. Until then, all you need to do is stay open, look for cues, and focus on your own journey. As you begin to know yourself more, you'll instinctively know the best way to help others. Sometimes that might mean reaching out. Other times it might mean stepping back. These learnings are a big part of what makes Bold Freedom so special. This journey begins with you, but there's no limit to where it can end.

~

STEP 10 REFLECT AND KNOW

The best way to learn about yourself (and, in time, help others) is to pay attention to how you're travelling. Think of Bold Freedom like a big road trip and your calendar like a map. You know which direction you're heading, but you still need to navigate as you go. This is unchartered territory, after all! Bold Freedom has quarterly check-in points, so you can fine tune your plan as the path becomes clear. Of course, you can pivot daily or weekly, but try to save any big detours until the end of the quarter. You need to travel far enough to see if you are going in the right direction, and you can't do that if you're constantly changing. Here are some tips to help you find the smoothest route to your destination.

- **Q1:** Stick to your roadmap as much as possible in the first leg of your journey. In the last week of Q1, sit down and review your travels. Are you heading in the right direction? Does your vision still hold up? Review your goals, refine your plan, and update your calendar as needed. As you go through this process, remember to keep your "why?" in mind. Give yourself time to complete this process. A whole weekend is ideal. Treat it like you're planning a party. This is a time to celebrate you and how far you've already come!

- **Q2:** Repeat the process in the last week of Q2. You should be halfway to your big goal by now. How are you travelling? Do you have enough time? Can you slow down, or should you speed up? If you're tempted to change direction here, there could be a "why behind the why". Get clear on this now before you begin the next quarter.

- **Q3:** Review again at the end of Q3. Have you achieved all your quarterly goals? Are you on target to meet your annual goal? Remember we talked about how businesses tend to cruise all year, then surge home in the final quarter? By following the Bold Freedom method, you should progress steadily. However, if you need to make a big final effort (which is more likely if you've changed your goals), now's the time to map it out.

- **Q4:** Hopefully you've hit your goals by the end of Q4. Remember to celebrate your success! You should be feeling healthier, happier and more aligned, but your journey doesn't need to end here. There's always further you can go – always room to grow and evolve. Take time to reflect on your progress and start thinking about what's next. What's your plan for the new year? What big goals would you love to achieve next? Begin the method all again and get ready to up-level your life!

~

To become a master of anything, you must practice. Keep practicing health and happiness every day. Make time to continue learning about yourself – because, after all, you are always changing. Be kind, curious and compassionate, and focus on what really matters. Don't waste time worrying about trivial things or comparing yourself to others. Remember, we are all different. We all want different things. The more you tap into what you REALLY want, by accessing your Vijnanamaya Kosha, the more you'll realise it's all possible. Intuition and consistency is all you need. All your dreams are within reach.

It's been an honour to guide you through the Bold Freedom method. I hope you've enjoyed learning the art of Ayurveda and how to integrate your body and mind. Most of all, I hope you've found more time to live well.

Before you close this book for now, think about how far you've come. Imagine how your life would look if you'd never discovered Bold Freedom. You should be incredibly proud of your journey and the positive energy you've created. If you'd like to pay this energy forward, please mention the Bold Freedom method to anyone you think is ready to receive it. You'll know in your heart who that may be, and when the time is right. Until then, stay healthy and happy – and always live boldly free!

4 | Enjoy the practice

ABOUT THE AUTHOR

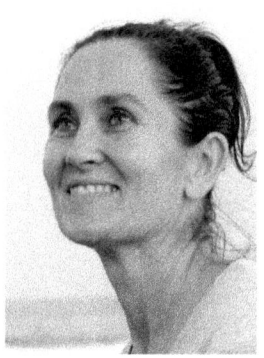

Ayurvedic Medicine Practitioner (Naturopath), Myotherapist, Public Health Researcher.

Lover of kayaking and bushwalking in Tasmania, bike riding, Yoga and wholefood cooking.

Lesley trained as an Ayurvedic medicine practitioner in Australia for three years with master Ashtavaidyan A.N. Narayanan Nambi MD (Ayu) Kerala India, Ray Noronha, Dr Vishnu Pillai and Dr Bosco Paul.

Lesley learnt languages and kitchen pharmacy from immersion into many Asian cultures and traditions while living in Singapore, Malaysia, Indonesia, China and India. She's lived in cities, regional and rural towns in Australia, which added invaluable experience about human behaviour and a variety of health conditions. With a caring practical approach over ten years, Lesley has helped people from as young as two to ninety three years of age with a broad range of health conditions. From digestive issues and acne, to insomnia and Parkinson's disease, Lesley works with the human body's natural ability to heal deeply and sustainably.

Since 2001 Lesley has co-authored a cook book (out of print), held workshops in Ayurvedic Theory, Cooking and Massage, completed trainings in Health Coaching and Aged Care, consulted and cooked for commercial kitchens and events and established two health clinics in Australia. She's been a rural fire fighter and created two start ups, which aimed to provide people with healthier product options for the home, and to connect well-being professionals with eachother for mentoring and resource sharing. Lesley founded AyurBotanicals clinic and herbal range and hosted the Radical Ayurveda Podcast. After a few years the businesses were streamlined through the central hub of Tiny House Ayurveda.

In 2021, Lesley made sure all her patiens and students were referred to the best care and wound down the business. She went on to support her peers in the health sector and the people who rely on the health system, by affecting positive change as a public health researcher at Torrens University Australia. She lives in a semi off grid tiny house in Tasmania, Australia and makes pure beeswax candles for local stores in her spare time.

Bold Freedom has been re-released so you can uplevel your wellbeing and bring your creations into the world.

MY NOTES:

MY NOTES:

MY NOTES:

www.ingramcontent.com/pod-product-compliance
Lightning Source LLC
Chambersburg PA
CBHW062040290426
44109CB00026B/2683